Peak Performance Fitness

"This encouraging and intelligently written book belongs in all wellness collections and in public and academic libraries that support health-related or physical education curricula. Anyone who is serious about physical fitness or who works in the field should read this well-conceived book."

—Library Journal

I dedicate this book to the four most important forces in my life:
My parents—thank you and I love you;
My husband, Jim—you are the best thing that ever happened to me;
God, for giving me the focus and the vision.

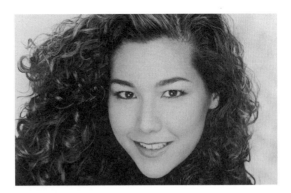

Jennifer Rhodes

Jennifer Rhodes has a master's degree in physical therapy from Columbia University and is the director of J.D. Rhodes Wellness and Fitness Consulting, works as an orthopedic physical therapist, and is an instructor at Equinox Fitness Clubs in Manhattan. Few authors combine such credentials and knowledge of the literature with practical experience as a personal trainer and aerobics instructor. She uses the techniques taught in her book to help thousands of clients rehabilitate themselves, prevent future injuries, and improve their overall health. She also conducts regular workshops on health and fitness.

Jennifer Rhodes is on the advisory board of *Jump* magazine, writes abstracts and reviews for the *APTA Journal,* contributes frequently to various national magazines (*Allure, Fit, Details,* and *Family Circle*), and has appeared as a health/fitness expert on numerous television shows on the Food Network, Fox Television, and ESPN 2. Jennifer is a member of the Sports Orthopedic Section of the American Physical Therapy Association, the American College of Sports Medicine, and the National Strength and Conditioning Association.

Ordering

Trade bookstores in the U.S. and Canada, please contact:

Publishers Group West
1700 Fourth Street, Berkeley CA 94710
Phone: (800) 788-3123   Fax: (510) 528-3444

Hunter House books are available at bulk discounts for textbook course adoptions; to qualifying community, health care, and government organizations; and for special promotions and fund-raising. For details please contact:

Special Sales Department
Hunter House Inc., PO Box 2914, Alameda CA 94501-0914
Phone: (510) 865-5282   Fax: (510) 865-4295
E-mail: ordering@hunterhouse.com

Individuals can order our books from most bookstores or by calling toll-free:

(800) 266-5592

Peak Performance
FITNESS

Maximizing Your Fitness Potential Without Injury or Strain

Jennifer Rhodes, M.S.PT

Hunter
House
PUBLISHERS

Hunter House Inc., Publishers
PO Box 2914
Alameda CA 94501-0914

Library of Congress Cataloging-in-Publication Data
Rhodes, Jennifer.
    Peak performance fitness : maximizing your fitness potential without injury or strain / Jennifer Rhodes.
      p. cm.
    Includes bibliographical references and index.
    ISBN 0-89793-296-X
    1. Physical fitness. 2. Wounds and injuries—Prevention. I. Title.
RA781.R48 2000
613.7'1—dc21   00-057241

Project credits
Cover Design: Peri Poloni
Photographs: Robert Vance Blosser
Illustrations: Christine A. Schaar
Model: Jennifer Rhodes, M.S.PT
Book Design and Production: Jinni Fontana
Developmental and Copy Edit: Jeff Campbell
Proofreader: John David Marion
Indexer: ALTA Indexing
Production Manager: Keri Northcott
Graphics Coordinator: Ariel Parker
Acquisitions Editor: Jeanne Brondino
Associate Editor: Alexandra Mummery
Editorial Intern: Martha Benco
Publicity Manager: Sarah Frederick
Marketing Assistant: Earlita Chenault
Customer Service Manager: Christina Sverdrup
Order Fulfillment: Joel Irons
Publisher: Kiran S. Rana

Printed and Bound by Publishers Press, Salt Lake City, Utah
Manufactured in the United States of America

9 8 7 6 5 4 3 2 1   First Edition   00 01 02 03 04

Table of Contents

Table of Contents

Table of Contents

Table of Contents

Table of Contents

Important Note

The material in this book is intended to provide a safe, effective exercise program. Every effort has been made to provide accurate and dependable information, and the contents of this book have been compiled through professional research and in consultation with medical professionals. However, always consult your doctor or physical therapy practitioner before undertaking a new exercise regimen or doing any of the exercises or suggestions contained in this book.

The author, publisher, editors, and professionals quoted in this book cannot be held responsible for any damage, injury, or other adverse outcome that may result from applying the information in this book in an exercise program carried out independently or under the care of a licensed trainer or practitioner. If you have questions concerning the application of the information described in this book, consult a qualified and trained professional.

Foreword

Joan E. Edelstein
Director, Program in Physical Therapy
Columbia University

Fitness is for everyone. The explosion of recent research confirms that children, adolescents, Generation Xers, Baby Boomers, and yes, even retirees can and do improve their physical and emotional health through exercise. More important than laboratory and clinical studies is the personal evidence that one accumulates after starting a consistent exercise program. Distances seem shorter, stairways fly beneath your feet, and clothing is looser. Friends start commenting on how well you look and the mirror becomes friendly. Self-confidence soars, for you have learned how to use precious time effectively and you can see the results yourself.

The key to reaping all these benefits is knowing how your body functions and its signals that indicate when it is overstressed. This knowledge, together with an understanding of the elements of an individualized fitness program, is what makes *Peak Performance Fitness* so special. Rather than relying on equipment that too often becomes a costly clothing rack, Jennifer Rhodes has carefully selected the most efficient exercises that utilize ordinary household items and inexpensive weights and has provided a logical method of exercising for people of all skill levels to follow.

It is a source of great pride for me to introduce you to Jennifer and her work. She has more than fulfilled her potential as a dynamic student and an outstanding graduate of Columbia University's Program in Physical Therapy. Jennifer combines wisdom honed by her classroom and laboratory studies and clinical experience in our rigorous graduate curriculum with her love of movement. Her success in her multifaceted professional practice reflects her enthusiasm, energy, and education. She is able to describe anatomy in simple, accurate terms so that everyone can appreciate how each exercise relates to a particular part of the body. Jennifer's breezy, easy-to-read style conveys a wealth of insights into exercise physiology, biomechanics, kinesiology, and sports psychology. Amidst today's mountains of exercise manuals, videotapes, and infomercials, *Peak Performance Fitness* is distinctive for its scientifically sound approach that can lead you to a lifetime of good health.

I am certain that you will enjoy *Peak Performance Fitness,* and I sincerely hope you will use it as your guide to achieving the wonderful advantages that a carefully structured exercise program can bring to you.

Chapter 1

Any Injury Can Be Prevented Through Healthy Alignment

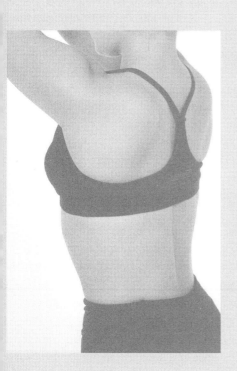

Janet, a 42-year-old dentist, had been active most of her life; she enjoyed running, bicycling, and aerobic classes. For 2 or 3 years, though, she had noticed that it had become increasingly difficult to raise her right arm above chest level without pain and that by the end of the day her right hand felt numb. She had stopped running because of chronic knee pain, which was exacerbated by prolonged sitting and going up and down stairs. And for the first time in her life, she had chronic low back pain. Janet was frustrated because, although she had joined a gym in an attempt to get into better shape, she felt that her new weight lifting routine had actually made her pain worse.

"Jennifer, I'm so tired. It seems like the more that I try to help myself, the more I end up hurting myself. I'm scared because it is really affecting my ability to take care of my patients."

I explained to Janet that it was not what she was doing that was harming her body but how she was performing these activities. To get better, she needed to make permanent changes in how she used her body in every aspect of her life—especially at work. Encounters with patients like Janet are the reason I wrote this book. I realized that most of my patients' injuries were the result of simple malalignment issues that had degenerated over the years into serious medical problems. A malalignment is when a body part (i.e., neck, shoulder, knee) is held or used in a way for which it was not designed. For example, sitting hunched over a desk or always carrying a heavy bag on the same shoulder would predispose an individual to low back and shoulder malalignments respectively. Sometimes the term misalignment is used to describe this condition, but I prefer malalignment because it's more accurate and is the term you might encounter from a doctor or in a medical setting. I felt that had I been able to intervene in my patients' lives earlier and given them the tools to correct their postural flaws they would have never suffered a serious injury. What follows is the revolutionary approach I used to empower Janet and thousands of others to improve their alignment for a lifetime of health and fitness.

This Is Not Your Usual Fitness Book

This book is different from most fitness books because it is not about giving you sleek thighs, tight buns, or big biceps. This book is about taking responsibility for your health, improving your alignment to prevent injuries, and making permanent changes in how you exercise so that you maximize results. This book will change the way you look at your body and the way you move, and it will encourage you to exercise for health and better functioning, not aesthetics.

I am a licensed physical therapist, personal trainer, aerobics instructor, and a student of the movement arts—such as yoga, the works of Joseph Pilates, and the Alexander Technique—and my approach is an eclectic one. I am not a student of any particular school of thought, I

am a student of results. *Peak Performance Fitness* combines the mindfulness of the movement arts with exercise physiology.

Most injuries can be prevented. Musculoskeletal (muscle and skeletal) injuries are the result of poor alignment, which puts undue stress on certain structures. If motions are repeated in poor alignment, they push the muscles and joints to the point of failure—and then you have an injury. Prolonged repetitive stress can occur when you have poor alignment while sitting in front of a computer, running, or doing heavy lifting. In Janet's case, her profession as a dentist required her to sit for long periods of time hunched over with her right arm elevated in an awkward position. Combined with her poor posture and muscle weakness, this predisposed her to the neck, shoulder, knee, and low back problems she described when she first came to see me.

How This Book Is Structured

The *Peak Performance Fitness* program begins with a self-evaluation in **Chapter 2,** "Your Unique Alignment," which will identify your unique posture, and then we proceed through five workouts designed to target specific problem areas that are meant to be integrated into a weekly routine. The chapters are paired so that the first chapter explains why certain alignments predispose an individual to particular injuries, while the second chapter is the "solution" to those alignment problems.

Chapters 3 and 4 discuss why low back pain is a vicious cycle that can be broken and present an exercise program designed to prevent low back pain and flatten your stomach.

Chapters **5 and 6** discuss the common causes of knee pain and describe a program that addresses lower extremity problems, such as those in the hips, knees, and ankles.

Chapters **7 and 8** explain the causes of most neck and shoulder injuries and present an exercise program designed to increase the power and endurance of your postural muscles.

Chapters **9 and 10** address the importance of flexibility and proper breathing in the prevention of injuries and present the extensive flexibility training solutionthat will help you improve the fluidity of your movements.

Chapters **11 and 12** build the case for the importance of cardiovascular exercise and show you how to develop your own regular cardiovascular training program. Chapter 12 also includes an extensive walking program that will maximize your cardiovascular training sessions.

Finally, in **Chapter 13,** I show you how to put it all together to develop an exercise and fitness routine that fits your goals and schedule and will ensure success on your journey to a healthier life.

The Three Main Types of Exercisers

The programs in this book can help anyone, but they should be approached somewhat differently depending on your current physical condition, experience, and goals. See which of the following groups you fall into and use the book accordingly.

New exercisers or those who have been on sabbatical—This book will teach you the basic breathing, alignment, and strengthening techniques you will need to build a strong exercise foundation.

Regular exercisers—The prescribed programs for each body part should replace your current strengthening program. In time, if you desire, and only after you can execute the program in perfect form, you may add back some of your current exercises. If some of your current exercises are included in the program, please do not skip that section on the assumption that you already know the exercise. I promise that you have never examined the exercise the way we will. Please continue your existing cardiovascular program (running, bicycling, walking), but begin to integrate the techniques in this book as you learn them. The key to the program is efficiency and consistency of movement.

Elite athletes—Just as with the regular exerciser, this program should replace your current strengthening program. It is an excellent supplement to any athlete's program and will boost your performance while preventing injuries. For you, the key is to maximize your strengthening time so that you can spend more time focusing on your sport. You should continue with any existing cardiovascular, interval, plyometrics, or other specialized training. However, begin to employ the alignment techniques as you learn them. The more efficient your movements, the less energy you will use and the more energy you will have available to win!

A Few Things to Buy

The following items are necessary for the execution of this program. Some of these you may already own, but if not, you will need to buy them.

■ *Portable mirror*—This is available from your local hardware store and should cost approximately twenty dollars. The ideal size is approximately 1 foot by 4 feet. It is important that the mirror be sturdy enough so that you can lie it on its side on the floor as well as stand it upright.

■ *One 20-pound or two 10-pound adjustable ankle weights*—These are available from your local sporting goods or medical supply store. The weight should consist of removable metal rods with a total weight of 10 or 20 pounds. It is very important for the weight to be adjustable, so that it can be changed to match your appropriate fitness level, which will evolve through time. Check to make sure that there is an adjustable strap that allows you to wrap the weight securely around both your ankle and your wrist.

■ *Floor*—Most of the exercises are done on the floor. Clear some space, designate it your exercise area, and keep it permanently clear from clutter. This is the area where you will store your equipment (such as weights, mirror, and three-ring notebook).

■ *An upright, sturdy, armless chair.*

■ *Towels*—You will need a large towel to lie on and a small one for the exercises.

■ *Six-foot rope*—This is used during flexibility training. It can be purchased from a hardware store, or you can substitute a bathrobe belt.

■ *A water bottle*—You should drink 4 ounces of water for every 15 minutes you exercise.

■ *Three-ring notebook and pen*—You need to keep track of your program and your progress. This will be discussed further in Chapter 13.

Constant Companion

This book should be your constant companion over the next couple of months as you learn the various programs. You want it handy so you can reference the various alignment cues throughout your day. We begin by refining your movements while you exercise, but eventually this improved alignment should permeate every aspect of your life, so that you are always aligned and moving with maximal efficiency. Feel overwhelmed? That is okay. We will start small and then build. Anyway, most people say that the integration happens seamlessly and often unconsciously.

One final note: I am very alarmed by today's approach to exercise and health. We are a society that loves quick fixes. When it comes to your health, there are no instant solutions, and you should be wary of anyone who promises you one. The human body is the world's most perfect machine. If you respect your body and take care of it, it will take care of you. Being healthy is your responsibility. This book is merely a tool. It is meant to introduce you to your body, develop a fitness program unique to your alignment, and teach you how to carry this movement pattern into all aspects of your life. Taking responsibility for your health is a lifelong commitment, and this book will help. There are no quick fixes.

Chapter 2

Your Unique Alignment

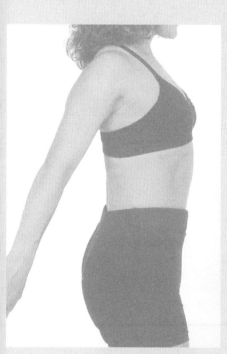

Your body today is the result of the various stresses (both good and bad) that have been placed on it throughout your life. These stresses have affected your posture, muscle lengths, joint position, and movement patterns and created an alignment that is unique to you. When you develop injuries, they are usually in areas of your body that have been weakened over time from repetitive stress. You are only as strong as your weakest link, and knowing your personal alignment helps you identify those weak links. Your alignment is the position you tend to return to, and it will predict how you will attempt to cheat, or compensate for your weak links, during the exercises. Our goal is to refine your movement patterns so as to strengthen your weak links, stretch the tight structures, and increase the efficiency of your movement—and, by doing all of these things, prevent future injuries and develop a more healthy alignment. The following postural evaluation (PE) will help you customize a program that addresses your unique alignment.

Time to Get Undressed

To determine your unique posture, you need to get undressed and stand in front of a mirror in your undergarments. You must be able to see yourself from head to toe. Many clients are initially uncomfortable with this aspect of the evaluation. I am often asked, "Can't you see my posture through my clothes?" The answer is no. Every bone and muscle must be visible so that you can determine if they are in the correct position.

What also often happens in the clinic during this portion of the evaluation is that clients begin to apologize to me about their bodies. These comments are always unsolicited. Clients will say, "Normally, I don't have these love handles. I've just been so busy with work." Or, "I think I have my mother's thighs. Hers are big, too." My regular response is that my examination is about function, not aesthetics. I tell them that I am examining their alignment and am noting the position of each structure in relation to surrounding body parts. This is the same way you need to look at your body during the postural evaluation, from the viewpoint of a clinician. I also tell them that the definition of a healthy body is one that is flexible, strong, and moves in optimal alignment. You should focus your energies on this type of body, not on one based purely on aesthetics. Furthermore, you should be congratulating yourself, not criticizing yourself, during the postural evaluation. By learning the programs in this book, you are taking positive steps, in some cases the first ones, toward making permanent improvements in your health.

Once you have put on your clinician's hat, stand facing the mirror and record your observations in pencil on the Front Postural Evaluation sheet. Then turn to the side and record your observations on the Side Postural Evaluation sheet. You should have separate comments for the right and left sides of your body. There are additional Postural Evaluation sheets in Appendix B, which will be used for future evaluations.

Interpreting Your Postural Evaluation

The Postural Evaluation helps you determine what your primary malalignment issues are. These are the weak links in your body that precipitate an injury at either that body part or at a distant location as your body attempts to compensate for the malalignment. It is important that you remain attuned to these problem areas while exercising.

During the Front Postural Evaluation the first aspect examined is the head position. If your head is tilted right, left, front, or back, this indicates neck muscle tightness on the side where you are tilted. For example, if your head tilts right, it means your right neck muscles are tight. Long-term tightness in the neck region can set up an individual for a whole host of neck, shoulder, and jaw problems (as we will learn in Chapter 7). Most jaw problems are actually the result of poor neck alignment.

When examining your shoulders, you may notice an asymmetry from right to left. Many factors can precipitate this, such as hand dominance, carrying a heavy bag on the same shoulder, cradling a phone on the same shoulder, or poor alignment while at the computer. This, combined with forward-sloping shoulders, compromises the normal alignment of the neck, shoulders, and even the back, which will predispose an individual to conditions such as shoulder tendonitis or a herniated disc.

Unlevel hips can be the result of muscle tightness or a leg length discrepancy. The *Peak Performance Fitness* program is designed to reverse any muscle tightness you may have. Correction of any type of leg length discrepancy is beyond the scope of this book and should be addressed by a medical professional. To determine the cause of your hip malalignment, stand

Front Postural Evaluation

Body Part	Proper Alignment	Your Alignment
Head	Centered over neck and shoulders	☐ Centered ☐ Tilted right or left ☐ Note asymmetry of the jaw ☐ Head protruding forward
Shoulders	Level without any forward rounding	☐ Level ☐ Right or left higher ☐ Both elevated ☐ One or both shoulders sloping forward
Hips	Level	☐ Place hands on top of hips and check if one hip is higher
Knees	Both kneecaps level and facing forward	☐ Legs are straight ☐ Knees touch when feet are apart (knock-knee) ☐ When feet are together, knees are apart (bow-legged)
Feet	Inside arch looks like a small dome Feet are parallel	☐ Inside edge of foot flattens out (flatfoot) ☐ High arch ☐ Foot and toes turn out (duck-foot) ☐ Foot and toes point inward while standing (pigeon-toed)

in front of the mirror with your hands on top of your hips and note which one is higher. Then sit in a chair in front of the mirror with both feet flat on the floor. Again, place your hands on top of your hips and recheck your hip levels. If your hips continue to be uneven, then you have an issue that can potentially be helped through the *Peak Performance Fitness* program. However, if your hips even out, this means your malalignment is caused by a leg length discrepancy, and you need to contact a medical professional for further evaluation. A leg length discrepancy is not a serious medical issue and is usually the result of a short bone or inadequate knee motion. However, you want to consult a medical professional to ensure that the cause is correctly identified and treated properly.

When looking at your knee alignment, also note the tone and development of your thigh and calf muscles. Look to see if one leg is more muscular than the other or if the muscles on the same leg are equally developed. Any differences that you observe could hint at a long-standing muscle imbalance that will predispose you to injuries (which will be discussed in Chapter 5).

We rarely look at our feet, which is a shame. Our feet directly connect us to the ground, and they have the greatest impact on our alignment. Continue to stand up straight when examining your feet in the mirror. This ensures you are seeing them while they are supporting your entire body weight. A healthy foot has a nice small dome for an arch. As we will learn in Chapter 5, having an arch that is too small or too big can predispose you to injury. Also note if your feet tend to turn in or out. This is often a compensation for hip inflexibility.

During the Side Postural Evaluation, keep in mind your Front Postural Evaluation malalignments and pay special attention to those areas. The side view clearly shows us how connected our body parts are. For example, bend and then hyperextend your knees so that the angle between the bones of the knee joint is greater than normal. Notice how this affects the position of your shoulders and low back. The reason this change occurs is because your body likes to be perfectly balanced. If anything throws the body off balance, it compensates appropriately. However, these compensations are often contrary to the way the body was designed, which results in excess wear and tear and ultimately in an injury.

Your spine has three main curves (see Figure 2.1). The major role of these curves is shock absorption. You have a slight forward curve of your neck, a backward curve of your upper back, and a forward curve of your lower back. A forward curve is called a lordosis, while

Side Postural Evaluation

Instructions: Stand with your left side near the mirror. Repeat the evaluation with your right side near the mirror.

Body Part	Proper Alignment	Your Alignment
Head	Ear over shoulder with slight curve forward of neck	☐ Chin held high ☐ Head protruding forward
Shoulder	Shoulder in line with hip	☐ Shoulder rounded forward ☐ Shoulder pulled back ☐ Marked rounding of upper back (kyphosis)
Abdomen	Entire abdomen is flat	☐ Flat ☐ Entire abdomen is protruding ☐ Upper abdomen is flat but lower portion protrudes
Knee	Knees straight	☐ Knee bent forward ☐ Knee bent backward
Hips	Slight curve in low back Hips in line with knee and shoulder	☐ Increased low back curve (lordosis) ☐ Flattened low back curve

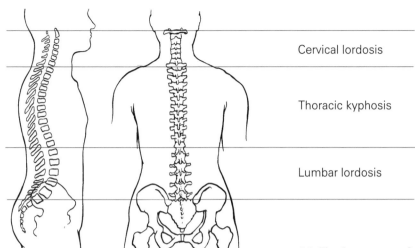

2.1. The three curves of the spine

Cervical lordosis

Thoracic kyphosis

Lumbar lordosis

a backward curve is called a kyphosis. Any increase or flattening of a curve will be compensated for in another curve, which will produce pain and make you vulnerable to injury. It is important to note the position and size of your curves.

Pay special attention to the size of your low back curve and the position of your buttocks. If you stand with an increased low back curve with your buttocks sticking out behind you like a table, then your abdominal muscles are stretched out and weak, while your low back and hip flexor muscles are tight. This issue will be addressed in greater detail in the next chapter. If you stand with a flattened low back curve and your buttock tucked under you, then your low back muscles are stretched out and weak while the muscles on the back of your leg are tight. These issues will also be addressed in the ensuing low back and flexibility chapters.

Figure 2.2 shows two common postural malalignments that illustrate how connected the body parts are. Compare your alignment to A and B and see if you match any of their typical injury patterns.

Typical injury patterns:

A. A person with this malalignment will have low back pain that is exacerbated

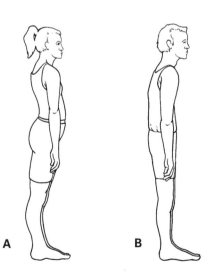

A   B

2.2. Two common postural malalignments

by prolonged standing but relieved by lying down with legs elevated. This person will also suffer from chronic knee pain and often describes himself or herself as a nonrunner because of "bad" knees.

B. This person will experience low back pain that is exacerbated by prolonged sitting but relieved by walking. He or she will also have problems lifting both arms above chest level without pain. These episodes of shoulder pain are usually worse after prolonged overhead-reaching activities, such as tennis or painting.

Both individuals will suffer from chronic neck pain, have headaches that radiate up the side of their skull, and feel like they cannot keep their head upright by the end of the day. Janet, our 42-year-old dentist from Chapter 1, was a combination of both malalignments. However, by becoming more aware of her alignment in all aspects of her life (at work, at the gym, and even while driving her car) and improving her strength and alignment by implementing the *Peak Performance Fitness* program, Janet was able to return to running and remain pain-free while treating her patients.

Cheating

You may not envision yourself as the cheating type, but as the Postural Evaluation should show you, you have been cheating unconsciously for a long time. By functioning in unhealthy alignment, you have robbed your body of the ability to move with maximal efficiency. The malalignments you noted are the primary ways you will attempt to cheat during the exercises. It is these old patterns that will predispose you to pain and injury. That is why it is vital to monitor your form via the mirror and written text cues during all the exercises. As your body learns the new efficient movement patterns from this program, maintaining healthy alignment will become easier and you will notice dramatic improvements in your strength, flexibility, and overall body awareness.

A Final Medical Note

If any of the following apply to you, please see a doctor before beginning *Peak Performance Fitness:*

- You have been in an accident (whether a motor vehicle accident or a fall).

- You feel numbness or tingling in your arms or legs.

- You have lost control of your bowel or bladder functions. This is a medical emergency, and you should seek immediate care.

- You are losing strength in your arms or legs.

- Your pain persists longer than 10 days and is accompanied by fever, nausea, or weight loss.

- You are pregnant.

- You have osteoporosis.

The above indications do not mean that you are not a candidate for the *Peak Performance Fitness* program. It is just advisable that you have yourself examined and cleared by a physician prior to beginning this program.

Chapter 3

Why Sit-Ups Don't Work

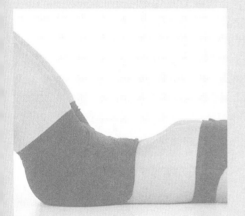

Rita, a 34-year-old attorney, had a history of chronic low back pain since college. She had tried everything from ab rollers to antigravity boots, but nothing alleviated her back pain. Historically, she would have an acute episode of low back pain once a year, which would be relieved by a couple days of rest. However, before she came to see me, her most recent episode had lasted for almost two months. Her biggest problem was severe low back pain that occurred whenever she stood for more than 10 minutes. This pain was relieved by lying down on her back with her legs elevated. Rita believed that the birth of her son seven months earlier might have contributed to her increased back problems. Prior to her son's birth, Rita had been going to the gym three times a week and rollerblading once on the weekends. However, since his birth she had not returned to the gym. She had instead been doing 100 sit-ups a day, which she thought may have actually made her back worse. During her first visit, she asked me why, despite all her efforts over the years, she was continuing to have low back problems.

The source of Rita's problem was weak abdominal muscles (abs). If you look at all of the fitness magazines today, you will see banners on the covers proclaiming, "Tight abs today," "Washboard abs in 5 minutes a day," and "Get rid of that belly." Do you ever wonder why people's abdominals remain weakened despite all these fitness magazines and despite all the focus on abdominal strengthening? Furthermore, if everyone is doing these abdominal exercises, then why do national statistics indicate that annually 15 to 20 percent of the population suffer from low back pain, which costs society approximately twenty to fifty billion dollars annually.

I'll tell you why! They are doing it all wrong.

In this chapter, we will examine the root causes of chronic low back pain, which is the result of the incremental stresses on the spine caused by poor posture and repetitive motions. Learning how to maintain good spinal alignment, not just during exercise but at all times, and strengthening the proper abdominal muscles (particularly, as we will see, the *transversus abdominis*) can reduce this stress and even eliminate it. I call these strengthening and alignment techniques "activating your core," an exercise that teaches your abdominal muscles how and when to contract to stabilize your spine. We will learn this technique in the next chapter, "The Low Back Solution." Done correctly, activating your core will improve how you look, prevent low back problems, and increase your athletic performance, but it takes a lifetime commitment. No matter what the magazines promise, there is no overnight cure.

You Have Been Exercising the Wrong Abdominal Muscle

Sit-ups will never work because they strengthen the wrong muscle and do not address the timing issue of when your abdominal muscles are activated. Your abdominals are comprised of four muscles (*rectus abdominis, external obliques, internal obliques,* and *transversus abdominis* (see Anatomy Lesson #3 on page 17). Sit-ups focus on strengthening the rectus

abdominis, and yet studies have shown that the muscle most important for healthy posture and the prevention of low back pain is the transversus abdominis. The transversus abdominis along with your low back muscles (and *fascial networks,* as we'll see in Anatomy Lesson #2 on page 16) form a corset around your midsection. When you tighten the transversus abdominis, it is like tightening the strings on the corset. Typical signs of a weak transversus abdominis are toned abdominals above the navel but a telltale bulge below it, an inability to hold in the stomach after a large meal or when gassy, and low back fatigue after prolonged standing or walking.

During Rita's postural examination, I found that though she was a slender woman, the area below her navel was protruding. She lamented that this was her problem area even before she had her son. She also felt that her abdominal region became very distended after a heavy meal. After performing a movement evaluation, I determined that Rita had a problem common to most low back patients. Not only did she have a weak transversus abdominis, but it was not activating early enough to splint her spine. As a result every time Rita moved her arms or legs, she was transmitting incremental stress to her low back. Once she had accumulated enough incremental stress, her low back would spasm and she would have an acute episode of low back pain. Her current episode of low back pain was severe for two reasons. One, the pregnancy had stretched and further weakened her already weak transversus abdominis muscle, and second, the physical demands of motherhood were subjecting her low back to even higher levels of stress than it had experienced in the past.

Why Timing Is Everything

As mentioned, Rita had a problem typical of many low back patients: an inability to control the timing of her abdominal muscles. Studies have shown that in people without low back pain the transversus abdominis is the first abdominal muscle to kick in whenever the arms or the legs move. For example, when hitting a tennis ball, the sequence of muscles being activated should be as follows: first the transversus abdominis, then the shoulder muscles, and finally the rest of the abdominal muscles. When kicking a ball, the sequence of muscles would be first the transversus abdominis, then the leg muscles, and finally the rest of the abdominal muscles. In patients with a history of low back pain, these studies have shown that the transversus abdominis reaction time is delayed. Instead of it kicking in first to help stabilize the spine, the transversus abdominis is activated after the arm or leg moves, which places undue stress on the spine. So, when patients with low back pain hit a tennis ball, the sequence of muscles is first the shoulder muscles and *then* the abdominal muscles, including the transversus abdominis. It's the same when kicking a ball: first the leg muscles and *then* the abdominal muscles, including the transversus abdominis.

As the above examples illustrate, low back pain is not only the result of weak muscles but also of bad timing. The relationship between the transversus abdominis and the spine is like that between the offensive linemen and the quarterback in football—both relationships require perfect timing by all parties involved. Imagine that the offensive linemen are the transversus abdominis and the quarterback is the spine. The linemen's job is to protect the quarterback from injury. If the linemen are not prepared, the quarterback gets hit or "sacked" by the opposing team. The more times the quarterback gets hit, the greater the chance of serious injury. So if your transversus abdominis is not prepared to protect your spine, your spine keeps getting "sacked."

A common misconception among low back pain victims is that it was one particular activity that produced their low back injury, when it was actually the result of many little mini-sacks or repetitive microtraumas to their spine. In fact, repetitive microtrauma is the cause of most injuries. If the body is used repeatedly in a way it was not designed to handle, it suffers undue stress. Over time, this stress or microtrauma adds up and the body breaks down. This breakdown can take many forms. In Rita's case, it manifested itself as low back pain. This is why learning to activate your core is so important. The term "core" refers to the region between the navel and spine, and contracting the transversus abdominis activates this area. Activating your core teaches your transversus abdominis how and when to prepare to protect your spine.

In an attempt to help themselves, low back patients like Rita do sit-ups, which primarily focus on strengthening the rectus abdominis, a muscle that has been shown *not* to be the primary stabilizer of the spine. Furthermore, studies have shown that sit-ups can actually further delay activation of the transversus abdominis. This is why low back pain cannot be treated without learning good transversus abdominis control.

Rita's Solution

Most people—excluding those who have had an acute trauma, such as a motor vehicle accident or a fracture—have low back pain due to repetitive stress on their spine. This is usually a combination of poor posture (sitting slumped over in front of a computer) or repetitive motion (poor lifting technique) with a deficient transversus abdominis. This was Rita's problem. After reviewing proper lifting techniques with Rita, I placed her on the Low Back Solution, which taught her how to activate her core. At the conclusion of a 12-week program, Rita was completely free from back pain and felt that the "problem area" below her navel was disappearing.

What follows is a more in-depth discussion of your low back and how it functions. This knowledge will further enhance your exercise sessions.

Anatomy Lesson #1: The Spine

Your spine is a truly amazing structure. It consists of thirty-three bones (called *vertebrae*) stacked on top of one another (see Figure 2.1). Your spine extends from the base of your skull to your tailbone. As you may have noticed, your spine is simultaneously mobile and supportive. It allows you to bend over and pick up a twenty-dollar bill off the street, stand in line to buy a movie ticket, reach for the popcorn box, and sit upright in the theater during the movie.

How Does Your Back Do It?

Your back has a lot of assistance to help it be so versatile. The vertebrae form the structural foundation of your spine, which is divided into four regions: *cervical* (skull to bottom of neck), *thoracic* (bottom of neck to midback), *lumbar* (midback to top of hips), and *sacral* (top of hips to end of tailbone).

Sitting between the vertebrae are fibrous cushions called *intervertebral discs*. They are the main weight-bearing structures of the spine; they act as shock absorbers, helping transmit the load of your body from vertebra to vertebra.

Connecting one bone to another are thickened cords of fibrous tissue called *ligaments*. They are not very elastic. Their job is to limit motion at the bone-to-bone connection, the joint. Ligaments exist all over your body wherever bones connect, and if put under undue stress, ligaments can get stretched, which is known as a sprain. You can sprain a ligament in your ankle as well as one in your back.

One of the primary jobs of the vertebrae is to protect the *spinal cord*, which is part of the central nervous system. Extending almost the entire length of the spine, your spinal cord passes information and orders from your brain—the president of Your Body, Inc.—to the rest of your body, and it even makes decisions locally to ensure that everything operates smoothly.

While your vertebrae provide a strong foundation, your back and trunk muscles enable you to move and breathe. These muscles are the workhorses of your body. Unlike muscles elsewhere, such as in your arms and legs, the muscles surrounding your trunk never rest! They work to help you breathe even while you are asleep. The muscles surrounding the spine come in many different shapes and sizes. Some run the full length of your spine, and some just go from one vertebra to the next. We will not go into much detail about the back muscles. However, remember that the muscles that run the length of your spine are connected to the abdominal muscles through something called...*fascia.*

WHAT'S A HERNIATED DISC?

A disc has two parts:

1. **Annulus Fibrosus**—thick outer band

2. **Nucleus Pulposus**—gel-like center

Imagine a jelly-filled doughnut. The annulus is the outer portion, while the jelly is the nucleus. If you press hard enough on the outer portion of the doughnut, the integrity of the doughnut will become compromised and the jelly will leak out. This is what happens when someone herniates a disc (see Figure 3.1). While this can happen anywhere in the spine, it is most typical in the neck and low back. When a disc pushes on the nerve, it can send shooting pains down either the arm or the leg. Medical treatment should always be pursued when this happens.

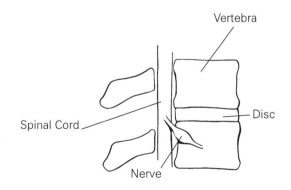

3.1. A healthy disc

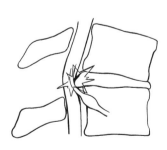

A herniated disc

Anatomy Lesson #2: "It's All Fascia to Me"

Fascia is the tough fibrous connective tissue that surrounds your muscles, organs, and nerves—pretty much everything. It is the web-like structure that holds everything in place. In the abdominal region, there are two important fascial networks: the *thoracolumbar fascia* and the *abdominal fascia* (see Figure 3.2). Because of the muscles attached to the fascia and its intrinsic stiffness, it plays a very important role in stabilizing the spine.

The thoracolumbar fascia is a thick fibrous sheet that is in the center of your low back. Your buttock, abdominal, and midback muscles all attach to it. The abdominal fascia is the union of the abdominal muscles with your main chest muscle (*pectoralis major*) and with the strong muscle (*serratus anterior*) that passes underneath both arms and along your rib cage. The serratus is usually well developed in boxers. It helps stabilize the shoulder complex so that you can do such things as throw, punch, and do push-ups.

These two fascial networks, along with your transversus abdominis muscle, are what form the "corset" around your midsection. The fascial networks are the body of the corset, and the transversus abdominis muscle is like the strings that tighten it. The stronger the strings, the tighter the corset. That is why "activating your core" stabilizes your spine and protects your back from the incremental strains that can ultimately lead to a low back injury. And that brings us back to the abs.

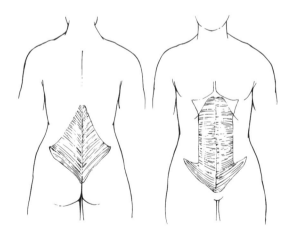

3.2. Thoracolumbar and abdominal fascia

Anatomy Lesson #3: What Exactly Are My Abs?

Your abdominals are comprised of four distinct muscles. The rectus abdominis is a broad strap of muscle whose fibers run vertically (see Figure 3.3). It originates at the pubic bone and connects to the rib cage and breastbone. The function of the rectus abdominis is to bend the trunk, and along with other abdominal muscles, it helps to stabilize the trunk during activities such as coughing and sneezing.

The external oblique is a flat muscle whose fibers run diagonally downward in the same direction as if you were putting your hands in your pockets (see Figure 3.4). You have one set of these on each side of your rectus abdominis. Each originates from ribs five through twelve and attaches to the front half of the hipbone (*iliac crest*), the *pubic bone*, and the abdominal fascia. Its function is to bend the trunk, rotate

WHAT'S A SIX-PACK?

When a person is very fit and you see the indentations of his or her abdominals, this is often referred to as a six-pack. What you are seeing is the junction of the connective tissue as it divides the rectus abdominis. The only way to get a six-pack is to use your abdominals as described in Chapter 4 and to have low body fat. You could have the world's strongest abdominal muscles, but if a layer of fat covers them, you won't see them. So the key to a six-pack is regular cardiovascular exercise, healthy eating, and efficient abdominal muscle use—not 300 sit-ups a day.

the trunk to the opposite side, and with the other abdominal muscles, help stabilize the trunk.

The internal oblique is a flat muscle whose fibers run from the bottom to the top (see Fig-

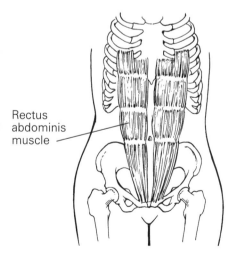

Rectus abdominis muscle

3.3. The muscle responsible for bending and stabilizing the trunk

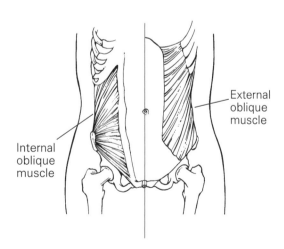

External oblique muscle

Internal oblique muscle

3.4. The muscles responsible for bending, rotating, and stabilizing the trunk

ure 3.4). It originates at the hipbone and the thoracolumbar fascia, the connective tissue it shares with the back muscles. It attaches to ribs ten through twelve and the line that runs down the middle of your abdomen called the *linea alba*. Its function is to bend the trunk, rotate the trunk to the same side, and act as a unique stabilizer of the spine, since it is connected to the back muscles via the thoracolumbar fascia.

Big Winner! Big Winner!

And the fourth abdominal muscle is...the *transversus abdominis* (see Figure 3.5)!

A flat muscle whose fibers run horizontally, it originates from ribs seven through ten, the thoracolumbar fascia, and the hipbone. It attaches to the linea alba and the abdominal fascia.

Its function is to stabilize the trunk by increasing the tension in the thoracolumbar and abdominal fascia. This muscle is the key to a healthy back and strong abdominals. In the next chapter, "The Low Back Solution," you will learn how to activate your core by turning on (triggering or utilizing) your transversus abdominis and your other muscles to develop a strong back and fit abdominals.

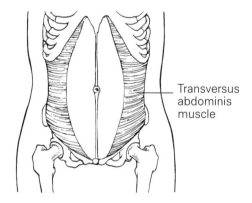

Transversus
abdominis
muscle

3.5. The primary muscle that stabilizes your spine by increasing the tension in the fascia

The Low Back Solution

The Painful Truth

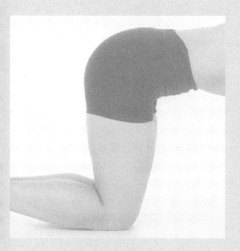

Sam, a 52-year-old artist, had chronic low back pain. His pain made him unable to stand for extended periods to paint, and he could no longer work out. This fact had him very depressed because he was still trying to lose the 15 pounds he had gained 5 years earlier after he quit smoking. When he came into my office, I told him the same thing I tell all my low back patients.

"Congratulations, you are now officially a low back patient! You will be a low back patient from now until forever. So in every aspect of your life, remember: *You are a low back patient.* Whether you are picking up a bag of groceries or brushing your teeth, you need to learn to use your body appropriately."

This is not what most people want to hear, but it is the truth. If you have chronic low back pain, you need strong abdominals and back muscles to protect and stabilize your back, and developing these is a lifetime commitment. Remember, if it were easy, no one would be struggling with this endemic problem.

Exercise Overview

The Low Back Solution is comprised of two main exercises, and each exercise has several levels. While these exercises are fairly simple, do not expect to go through the entire program in one session. It is vital that you "master" each level of each exercise before moving on. If this means you stay at Level 1 the first couple of sessions—so be it. Be honest with yourself and make sure that you are truly concentrating on the exercise. Steady focus and concentration early on will carry over to the rest of the exercise program and to other parts of your life as well.

Even when you have mastered both Low Back Solution exercises, you should always begin with Level 1. This will help you "wake up" your abdominals so that you will be aware of them during the rest of the exercises, and it will help center your energy.

Low Back Solution Exercise 1, which is done lying down, is the foundation of all other movements. As we've learned, studies have found that, in individuals with chronic low back pain, the transversus abdominis muscle failed to turn on early enough to splint the spine. No studies to date have shown conclusively which came first—the timing issue or the low back pain. But we do know that by improving the timing we can reduce low back pain and prevent future episodes.

Activating your core focuses on training your transversus abdominis, internal obliques, and low back muscles to activate properly and stabilize your spine. Maintaining this alignment and muscle control throughout your exercises ensures that your low back is protected and that your abdominals are being maximally strengthened. Eventually, the goal is for you to be able to activate your core in any position, whether running, lifting weights, standing in line at the grocery store, driving your car, or working at the computer. In time, this movement pattern will become automatic for you.

Once you can perform the sustained curl (Low Back Solution Exercise 1, Level 3) five times in good form, you are ready to proceed to the second abdominal strengthening series, Low Back Solution Exercise 2. Since you don't spend all of your time lying down, it is important that you learn how to activate your core in other positions. That is why this exercise series, which is done on all fours, is so important. These exercises remove the support of the floor and force your abdominals to stabilize your spine against an external resistance. You begin by activating your core while on your hands and knees (in the quadruped position). Once you have mastered activating your core in this position, the next step is lifting alternate arms. By reaching with your arms, you reduce your base of support and force your abdominals to work even harder to stabilize your spine. The next level teaches you how to keep your core activated while extending your leg, and eventually alternate arms and legs. This is more challenging than just the arms because your legs are longer and heavier.

Note: *None of these exercises should cause you low back pain. Muscle fatigue—yes. Pain—no. If you feel pain, check your form. If the pain continues, return to activating your core in the quadruped position and attempt the next level in a few weeks when you are stronger.*

What to Wear

When you do these exercises, the entire back and abdominal region *must* be exposed. If you are a man, do them with your shirt off. If you are a woman, perform the exercises in shorts and either an athletic bra or your regular bra. Being this exposed may feel a little awkward at first. That is all right. You will become more comfortable with your body as you build your exercise program. Remember, the human body is the most perfect machine. These machines come in all shapes and sizes, and they are all beautiful. The goal of this program is to fine-tune your machine, and you need to see it to know if it's working properly.

Equipment Checklist

- A mirror laid on its side on the floor next to you so you can watch your form.

- A towel to lie on. (The towel is optional; the mirror is not.)

NOTE: *If you are having shooting pain down either or both legs, please see a physician before performing this program. Also, if you have lost control of your bowel or bladder functions since the onset of your low back pain, please seek medical attention immediately.*

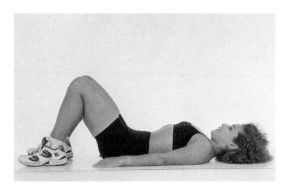

Starting position

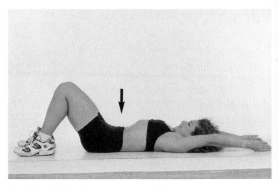

Level 1: Activating your core with arms up

Low Back Solution Exercise 1

Level 1: Activating Your Core with Arms Up

1. Lie on your back with both knees bent, feet on the floor.

2. Reach arms straight overhead to lift the rib cage upward toward your head.

3. Keeping the arms overhead:

   A. Take a deep breath in.

   B. As you exhale, pull your navel in (as though you were zipping up a tight pair of pants) and press your low back into the floor. This motion activates your core, the region between your navel and your spine.

   C. Hold this position for 10 seconds while breathing normally and then relax.

Check to make sure you are not using your legs to push your lower back into the floor. This is a common mistake that defeats the purpose of the exercise.

4. Repeat 3A to 3C five times. Watch the movement of your navel in the mirror.

Check to Make Sure:

- Neck is long and chin is tucked in.

- Back of shoulders are relaxed onto the floor.

- Chest is open.

You Should Feel Work Going on In:

- Your abdominals, especially the area below your navel.

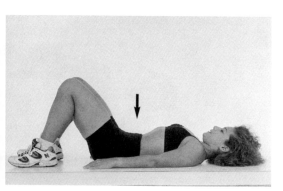

Level 2: Activating your core with arms down

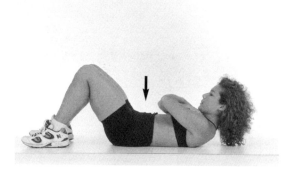

Level 3: The sustained curl

Level 2: Activating Your Core with Arms Down

Once you are able to keep your navel in for 10 seconds with normal breathing, progress to Level 2.

1. Repeat Level 1, steps 1 to 5, except keep your arms relaxed by your sides.

2. Repeat five times.

Level 3: The Sustained Curl

If you are able to execute Level 2 in good form for all 5 repetitions, then proceed to the sustained curl.

1. Lie on your back with knees bent and feet on the floor about shoulder-width apart.

2. Activate your core by pulling in your navel and keeping your back pressed into the floor, as you did in Level 2.

3. Cross your arms over your chest, lower your chin so it is on your chest, and now curl up so the backs of your shoulders are off the floor.

4. Hold this position for 10 seconds while breathing normally. Every time you exhale, pull your navel in more and more. Then relax your head back down onto the floor.

5. Repeat the sustained curl five times.

Check to Make Sure:

■ Shoulders are relaxed and back.

■ Chest is open.

■ No pushing through the legs.

You Should Feel Work Going on In:

■ Your abdominals, especially the area below your navel.

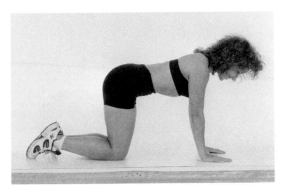

Quadruped position

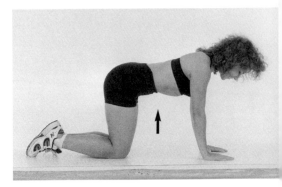

Level 1: Activating your core in quadruped

Low Back Solution Exercise 2

Level 1: Activating Your Core in Quadruped

1. Position yourself on all fours in the quadruped position.

2. Check yourself sideways in the mirror to ensure you have good alignment.

Does your back look arched? Scooped out? It should look flat, as in the photograph above. If it does not, then move your back up and down until it looks flat or almost flat. If you aren't able to assume the correct posture immediately, don't be discouraged. That's okay. It merely means that you have some tightness in your hips or back that needs to be addressed. The best way to stretch is to assume your best alignment. Always use the pictured alignment as your end goal and exercise in this position. If you do this, over a period of time your muscles will naturally elongate. We will address specific muscle tightness in Chapter 9, "Why You Should Never Stretch Before Exercising."

3. While in your best quadruped alignment, activate your core as you did in Exercise 1. Continue to use your breathing to help pull your navel in. Exhale as you pull your navel in and hold your navel in for 10 seconds while breathing normally. Repeat this ten times. Check yourself in the mirror to make sure there is no movement in your back.

Check to Make Sure:

■ Neck is long.

■ Shoulders are relaxed and away from your ears.

■ Back is flat and navel is in.

You Should Feel Work Going on In:

■ Your abdominals, especially the area below your navel.

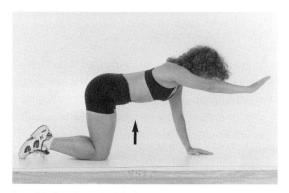

Level 2: Quadruped with alternating arms

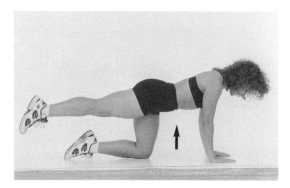

Level 3: Quadruped with alternating legs

Level 2: Quadruped with Alternating Arms

1. Activate your core in quadruped position.

2. Maintain your center, exhale, and reach with your right arm (don't worry about how high it goes). The moment your pelvis moves is the maximum height you should lift your arm.

3. Return the right arm to its original position. While staying activated through your core, reach with your left arm. Then return the left arm to its original position. The trunk should remain stable—no wobbling through your middle.

4. Repeat steps 1 to 3 thirty times, resting after every 10 lifts.

5. Every time you reach, exhale and pull your navel in.

6. You may notice that you can stabilize one side more easily than the other. This just lets you know what you need to work on. I have found with my patients that the weaker side is usually the side of their symptoms—is that true for you? If so, just work and focus on that side more.

Level 3: Quadruped with Alternating Legs

1. Activate your core in the quadruped position.

2. Maintain your center, exhale, and extend your right leg.

3. Return the right leg to its original position and then extend the left leg.

4. As you extend the leg, exhale and pull your navel in.

5. Repeat thirty times, resting between every 10 lifts.

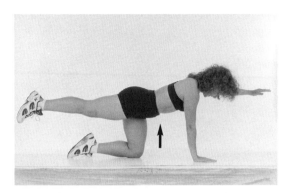

Level 4: Quadruped with alternating arms and legs

Level 4: Quadruped with Alternating Arms and Legs

Once you have mastered Level 3, move on to the final, fourth level.

1. Activate your core in the quadruped position.

2. Maintain your center, exhale, and reach with your left arm while extending your right leg.

3. Return your arm and leg to their original positions and then reach with the right arm while extending the left leg.

4. Repeat thirty times, resting between each 10 lifts.

FOAM ROLLER

In the clinic, this is an invaluable tool for helping patients find and develop better alignment. When lying on the roll, an individual should have the upper chest and spinal flexibility to place each vertebra flush on the roll.

How to use the roll:

- Lie on the roll and activate your core as discussed in the Low Back Solution Exercise 1 (Level 2) for 10 repetitions.

- While activating your core, tuck your chin and attempt to press the back of your neck onto the roll for 10 repetitions.

- Maintain this alignment and relax your shoulders back and down. Luxuriate in this position for a minimum of 5 minutes.

For ordering information, see Appendix D.

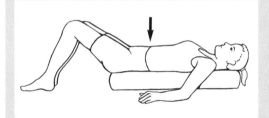

Chapter 5

Why Knee Pain May Be a Sign of a Foot Problem

When training for her first marathon, Alex, a 28-year-old sales representative, began experiencing severe knee pain that radiated from the sides of her knees to her hips. She also felt a "snapping" sensation at her hips and knees after longer runs. In the 3 weeks prior to her appointment with me, she had started having an "achy" pain in the back of her kneecap anytime she sat for more than ten minutes or whenever she went down stairs. Her knee pain had gotten so bad that she had stopped running altogether and was walking with a slight limp. Prior to beginning her marathon training, Alex's exercise routine had consisted of two 3–4-mile runs, two 5-mile runs, and a weekly step class. She told me her doctor had said that she had *patellofemoral pain* and *chondromalacia patellae.* I explained to her that these were medical terms meaning knee pain and kneecap pain, respectively.

Upon examination, I determined that Alex's problem was not her knees or her hips but her feet. Both of Alex's feet were extremely pronated (she had flatfeet). This malalignment in her feet was forcing her knees and hips to operate in a way that they were not designed for. The repetitive motion of running had simply magnified her foot malalignment at a faster rate. As a result, she was experiencing both hip and knee pain.

This is just one example of how compensation for a malalignment can create a weak link in the body and lead to an injury at the site. As in Alex's case, it is not uncommon for an individual with a foot malalignment to develop a knee problem, since we tend to first compensate for foot problems at the knee. If we let the problem progress without treatment, the knee problem will eventually become a hip and then a low back problem.

Lower extremity problems—those that involve your hips, knees, and ankles—can be among the most frustrating. Many of the patients I see injure themselves while attempting to get into better shape. Others have injuries related to their jobs or from the wear and tear of everyday life. The exercisers are frustrated because they were told to exercise to improve their health. They did what they were told, and now they are injured and can barely walk. In this chapter we will examine the common causes of lower extremity pain, which is often the result of poor bony alignment or a muscle imbalance. Since your lower extremities are your only connection to the ground, any compensation in them affects the rest of your body. However, by exercising in proper alignment, we can strengthen the weak muscles and stretch the tight ones, and thereby achieve maximum results and prevent injury.

Alex's Balancing Act

The problem Alex had with her knees is very common. Her pain was the result of two contributing factors, her bony alignment and a muscle imbalance. Bony alignment issues can be either congenital (you are born with them) or secondary to an injury (if you had, for instance, a hip dislocation or leg fracture as a child). Women are known for having a greater susceptibility to knee problems. Many researchers believe this is because of the width of women's hips. Women have wide hips by design—so that the birth canal in the pelvis is large enough for a baby to pass through—but the width of the hips changes the alignment of the knees and can predispose a woman to knee problems. This bony malalignment can come from the feet as well. For example, being flat-footed can predispose an individual to knee problems. This was how Alex's problems began. However, this was only half of her problem.

Alex also had a muscle imbalance. Not only is it important to maintain balance between opposing muscles, it is vital to maintain balance within a muscle group. No place is this clearer than in the thigh muscles (*quadriceps*). To maintain normal movement of the kneecap

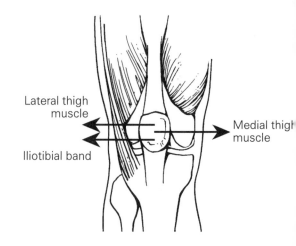

Lateral thigh muscle

Medial thigh muscle

Iliotibial band

5.1. Front view of the tug-of-war game at your kneecap

(*patella*), the medial thigh muscle (*vastus medialis oblique*) needs to balance the lateral thigh muscle (*vastus lateralis oblique*). In addition, a fibrous structure called the *iliotibial band* extends from the top side of the hip and attaches to the side of the knee joint, which means it can exert pressure on the kneecap. If any of these get out of balance, you have a recipe for knee pain. Imagine two people in a game of tug-of-war over a ditch, with both pulling with all their might. This happens daily as your medial and lateral thigh muscles fight for control of your kneecap (see Figure 5.1). If both are equally strong, then the kneecap stays balanced. But what happens in the tug-of-war game if one person is stronger or if a second person is added at one end of the rope? Of course, the weaker person loses and is pulled into the ditch. This is what happens when the thigh muscles are imbalanced or when the iliotibial band tightens up. The result is that the kneecap is pulled laterally, producing pain.

WHY SEATED KNEE EXTENSIONS ARE HARMFUL

Seated knee extensions are the worst exercise for your knees. As discussed, the cause of most knee pain is an irritation on the back of the patella. During seated knee extensions, the maximum force from the weight occurs when your patella is least able to disperse the load. As a result, this exercise grinds the patella into the femur and will exacerbate any underlying knee problem.

The iliotibial band can tighten up for many reasons. The two most common are overdoing an activity that your body is not strong enough to perform (such as running 6 miles when you had previously been running 3) and pronated feet. As a result of overtraining and her pronated feet, Alex's iliotibial bands had tightened and caused her kneecap to be pulled sideways, which had been described by her doctor as a laterally tracking patella. Your kneecap is designed to move in a C-shaped path or tracking pattern (see Figure 5.2). Tracking describes the path that the kneecap travels as you bend and straighten your knee. When your knee is straight, the patella is floating at the top and outside edge of the knee joint. As you bend your knee, it moves downward and in, and then it moves downward and out. Healthy patella tracking is when the patella adheres to this path much like a train on a railroad track. However, when the patella deviates from this path because of a muscle imbalance or tight iliotibial bands, as in Alex's case, pain ensues.

An improperly tracking patella is problematic for two reasons. First, the back of the kneecap and the front of the thighbone are specially

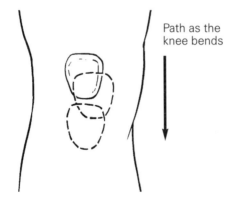

Path as the knee bends

5.2. Healthy patella tracking

reinforced with cartilage for shock absorption, but certain areas are more reinforced than others. When the kneecap deviates from its normal path, it rides on the less-reinforced areas, which can become inflamed and irritated, thereby exposing the knee joint and kneecap to repetitive stress or microtrauma. It is this repetitive microtrauma that wears away the knee cartilage and can, over time, produce arthritis. Second, when the patella is not riding in its normal path, it is less stable, making the person more prone to *subluxations* of the kneecap. A subluxation is when the kneecap pops completely off its path and then pops back in. If you bend and straighten your knee often and quickly (such as while running and biking) in this deviated pattern, you will soon develop a full-blown knee problem (as Alex's doctor correctly informed her, the common names for this problem are chondromalacia patella or patellofemoral syndrome). So you can see that the key to maintaining a healthy knee is to determine and address why your kneecap is not tracking properly.

As a result of her injury, Alex had some general weakness in both lower extremities. After being fitted with a pair of orthotics and performing the exercises in Chapter 6, "The Lower Extremity Solution," for 12 weeks, Alex resumed her marathon training and was free of pain. Realizing that prevention was key, Alex made the Lower Extremity Solution a permanent part of her twice-weekly strengthening program.

Why Exercise Your Feet?

Alex was very surprised that I had her exercise her feet. Did you know that when walking you are transmitting approximately 115 to 120 percent of your body weight to your lower extremities? If you are a 130-pound individual, each foot receives 150 pounds of pressure every time you put your foot down. And what do you think helps absorb all of this stress? Bones, yes. Ligaments, kind of. But mostly, your muscles!

Basic gait (that is, walking) can be divided into three distinct phases (see Figure 5.3). The first phase is when your heel strikes the ground and the foot is in a high arched position. Then as your weight is transmitted to the foot, the foot flattens out to absorb the shock. Finally, the foot returns to the high arch position as your heel rises and your toes push off the ground to propel you forward. Any deviation from this pattern predisposes an individual to foot injury.

Your Foot Type Determines Your Injury

Here's a test. Wet the bottom of your foot and step onto a piece of paper. Compare your footprint to those in Figure 5.4 and read about your foot type below.

If you have what is referred to as a floppy foot, a foot in which the arch flattens out when you stand, it is important that you have strong ankle and foot muscles. Because of your foot design, some of the bony stability has been lost, and for you to function without pain, your foot muscles need to act as dynamic stabilizers of

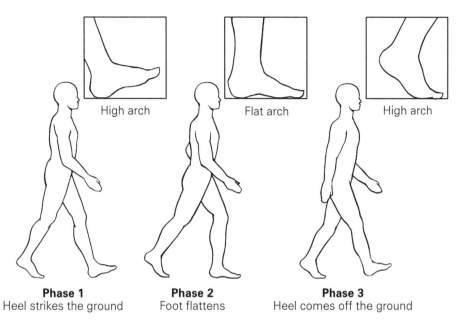

High arch   Flat arch   High arch

Phase 1
Heel strikes the ground

Phase 2
Foot flattens

Phase 3
Heel comes off the ground

5.3. The three phases of walking

your foot. Alex had a floppy foot. When her heel hit the ground, instead of landing in a high arched position, her foot was already flat. As her weight was transmitted to her foot, her foot flattened out even more, which forced her ankle muscles to work overtime

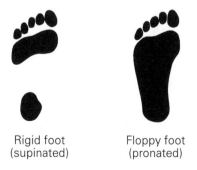

Rigid foot
(supinated)

Floppy foot
(pronated)

5.4. Determine your foot type

to absorb her weight. This also placed her knee in a vulnerable position. Then, when her heel came off the ground, instead of going into a high arched position, her foot continued to remain flat, which was not only inefficient but, again, forced her ankle muscles to be over-worked. For people with flatfeet, typical injuries include heel pain and essentially any *tendonitis* of the foot. Tendonitis literally means inflamed tendon and is the result of actual microtears in the tendon or at the muscle/tendon junction. This condition is another example of how repetitive microtrauma can result in an injury and can happen to any tendon whenever it is put under excessive stress. With flatfeet, the repetitive microtrauma is caused because the muscles are constantly being pushed beyond their normal limits as they try to stabilize the foot.

ORTHOTICS

Orthotics are shoe inserts that improve the alignment of your foot. Regardless of your foot type, if you are having any foot pain, it would be helpful for you to wear orthotics. There are two distinct foot types, the supinated and the pronated foot, and most of us fall somewhere between the two. If you have floppy or pronated feet, the orthotic will give you the support you need. If you have rigid or supinated feet, the orthotic will provide the shock absorption your foot lacks. Orthotics also improve the alignment of your knee, thereby reducing any patellofemoral problems you may be having.

There are two ways to obtain orthotics. You can either order a custom orthotic or purchase an over-the-counter (OTC) orthotic. A podiatrist, orthotist, or physical therapist can design an orthotic specifically for your foot. These typically cost anywhere from $250 to $400. A custom orthotic is excellent if you have a very specific, permanent alignment issue (such as a leg length discrepancy greater than a half inch) or are an elite athlete. However, the average person can experience a dramatic relief of symptoms with a much cheaper OTC orthotic. Clinically, most of my patients have had the greatest success with Spenco orthotics. For ordering information, see Appendix D.

For maximum benefit, the orthotic must be placed in a supportive lace-up shoe. The shoe must hold the orthotic in the proper position on your foot. Few sandals or loafers offer this type of support.

The flip side of the floppy foot is the rigid foot. The rigid foot stays in the high arch position (supination) during the entire gait cycle, and even when sitting. This type of foot also needs additional muscle strength because the bones are constantly locked in a stiff position with little or no shock absorption. Strong muscles can help to absorb some of the load. For people with supinated feet, typical foot problems are stress fractures, collapsed arches, and chronic ankle sprains.

Most of us have feet that fall somewhere between these two foot types. So the lesson of the day is…whatever your foot type, do your foot exercises!

More Anatomy!
The Lower Extremities

It is important to understand how all the parts of your lower extremities work to understand the problems originating from malalignment. The goal is for you to have a general understanding of the muscle groups and how they function so you can get the most out of your workout.

Your lower extremities have multiple functions. Their primary functions are to move you (walk, run, skip) and to connect you to the ground so your upper body has a stable base from which to operate. The second function is particularly important, since the lower extremities are the only things that connect you to the ground. Any malalignment or compensation in the lower extremities will throw off the rest of your body.

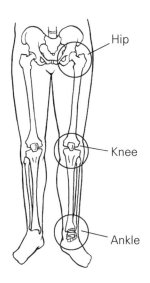

5.5. Joints of the lower extremity

The Hipbone Is Connected to the Thighbone, the Thighbone Is Connected to the...

Your lower extremities consist of many joints, but to simplify we will divide them into three main joints (see Figure 5.5). The hip joint is where your pelvis meets your thighbone (*femur*), while the knee joint is where your thighbone connects to your shinbones (*tibia* and *fibula*). The tibia is the larger bone. This is the one you hit on the coffee table in the middle of the night. The smaller bone is the fibula. Your ankle joint is where the shinbones meet your foot bone (*talus*). We will not go into great detail about the joints of the foot, due to their complexity. There are twenty-six bones, thirty-three joints, and a network of more than one hundred tendons, muscles, and ligaments—which basically means there are a lot of little bones in your foot and a lot of room for error.

Just as we did with the muscles of your abdomen, we will review the origin, point of attachment, and function of each group of muscles. Pay special attention to those muscles that cross two joints because when these groups get tight interesting things happen to your posture.

Anatomy Lesson #4:
The Hip Joint

Many motions occur at the hip, but they are all some permutation of four basic motions: hip flexion, hip extension, hip abduction, and hip adduction (see Figure 5.6).

Hip flexion is the motion of bringing your knee toward your chest. There are two muscles that flex your hip, the *iliopsoas* and the *rectus femoris* (see Figure 5.7). The iliopsoas muscle originates at your lumbar spine and the pelvis and attaches to the top outside portion of the thighbone. Its primary function is to flex the hip. The rectus femoris begins at the front part of the hip and attaches across the kneecap and onto the shinbone. Since the rectus femoris crosses two joints, it has two functions. It is responsible for both flexing the hip and extending (straightening) the knee.

Hip extension is the motion of lifting your leg straight back behind you. It is the motion a ballerina performs when executing an arabesque. The two muscles that help you perform this movement are the *gluteus maximus* and the *hamstrings* (see Figure 5.8). The gluteus maximus originates from different parts of the back of the pelvis and attaches to the back of the thighbone and the iliotibial band, which attaches to the top outside portion of the shinbone. The gluteus maximus is also a two-joint muscle. Its dual functions are to extend the hip and to assist in raising the trunk from a flexed position, such as standing up when you're bent over.

The hamstrings are actually three separate muscles. All three originate at the back of the pelvis (the part you sit on) and attach to both sides of the shinbone. As two-joint muscles, they extend the hip and flex (bend) the knee.

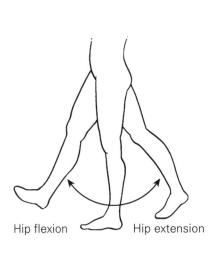

Hip flexion   Hip extension

5.6. The motions of the hip

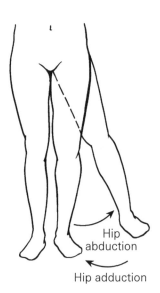

Hip abduction

Hip adduction

Tight hamstrings can predispose an individual to low back problems. Since the hamstrings originate at the pelvis, they can pull the low back into an unnatural position. If your postural evaluation in Chapter 2 revealed that you stand with a flattened lumbar lordosis (buttock tucked under), then you probably have tight hamstrings. Chapter 10 contains a program for increasing your flexibility.

Hip abduction is the motion of lifting your leg to the side. Several muscles comprise the abductor muscle group, and it's not necessary for you to know each individual muscle; instead, we will refer to the entire group as the abductors (see Figure 5.9). They originate at the back of pelvis and attach to the top outside portion of femur. The function of the abductors is to move the thigh away from the midline of the body.

Hip adduction is the motion of bringing your legs together, such as when crossing your legs. Like the hip abductors, the hip adductors con-

TIGHT HIP FLEXORS AND LOW BACK PAIN

Since the hip flexors connect your back to your legs, any abnormal motion of the hips will affect your back, and a tight iliopsoas will produce low back pain. If your postural evaluation in Chapter 2 revealed that you stand with an increased lumbar lordosis (your buttocks stick out really far), then you definitely have tight hip flexors. Also, the transversus abdominis weakness discussed in Chapter 3 usually coexists with tight hip flexors. Chapter 10 contains a flexibility program to address this tightness.

sist of many different muscles, and we will refer to them as a single group (see Figure 5.9). All of them originate at the pubic bone and attach to the inner thigh portion of the femur. The adductors move the thigh toward the midline of your body.

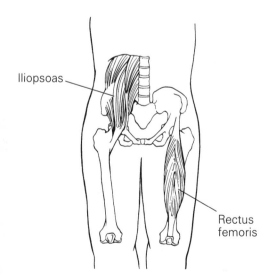

5.7. The muscles responsible for hip flexion

Iliopsoas

Rectus femoris

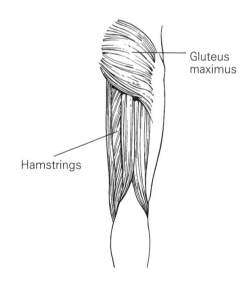

5.8. The muscles responsible for hip extension

Gluteus maximus

Hamstrings

A TIGHT BUTT

Clients are always asking for exercises to minimize this area. Fact—there is no such thing as a spot reduction exercise. As with the abdominals, you could have the firmest gluteus maximus in the world, but if a layer of fat covers it, no one will see it. A good cardiovascular and general strengthening program that addresses your overall fitness is the best way to get tight buttocks.

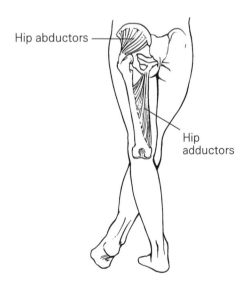

Hip abductors

Hip adductors

5.9. The muscles responsible for lifting your legs to the side and for bringing them together

Anatomy Lesson #5:
The Knee Joint

Two basic motions occur at the knee joint, extension and flexion. Extension is when you straighten the knee and flexion is when you bend the knee. Remember, a number of structures that cross the knee joint also cross either the hip or ankle joint. Weakness or inflexibility in any of these structures can affect you at multiple joints. The quadricep is a group of four muscles that extend or straighten your knee. Three of the four muscles originate at the top front portion of the thighbone and attach across the kneecap onto the shinbone. These three muscles are only able to perform knee extension, since their attachment sites are limited to the leg (see Figure 5.10). However, the fourth quadricep muscle, the rectus femoris, originates at the front of the hip and attaches across the kneecap onto the shinbone. Since it crosses the hip joint, the rectus femoris is able to both flex the hip and extend the knee.

The hamstring muscles, as discussed above, also act as knee flexors (see Figure 5.10). They are important stabilizers of the knee joint and can protect the knee from injury. The *gastrocnemius* is one of the two muscles that form the calf. It is the only one that flexes the knee. It begins at the bottom backside of the femur and attaches to the heel bone (*calcaneus*) via the *Achilles tendon*.

Why Have a Kneecap?

The main purpose of your kneecap, or patella, is to improve the mechanical advantage or pull of the quadriceps muscle. Without your kneecap you would have a hard time extending your knee. You would have difficulty walking, climbing stairs, and doing anything that required you to stand. In the clinic we often see postsurgical knee patients whose kneecaps are not moving because of scar tissue. We work hard to restore proper kneecap motion because without full motion these patients would never regain full strength in their quadriceps.

However, as discussed earlier, most individuals have knee pain because their kneecap has too much motion in the wrong direction. This can be readily corrected with proper alignment, balanced muscle strength, and good overall flexibility.

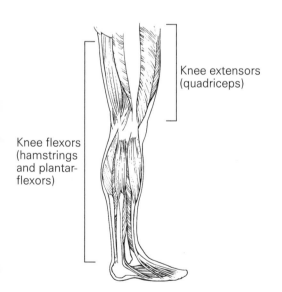

Knee extensors (quadriceps)

Knee flexors (hamstrings and plantar-flexors)

5.10. The muscles responsible for bending and straightening the knee

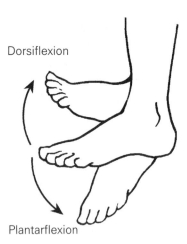

Dorsiflexion

Plantarflexion

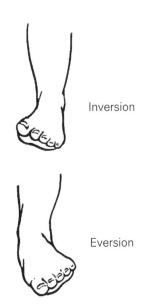

Inversion

Eversion

5.11. The motions of the ankle

Anatomy Lesson #6: The Ankle Joint

The bones of the ankle and foot have already been briefly discussed above. There are four basic motions that occur at your ankle: pointing your foot and toes (*plantarflexion*), flexing your foot and toes up toward your shin (*dorsiflexion*), bringing the inner edge of your foot upward (*inversion*), and bringing the outer edge of your foot upward (*eversion*) (see Figure 5.11).

The muscles that control these motions originate at the tibia and fibula and attach at different points on your foot. As elsewhere in your body, the origin and points of attachment determine the action each muscle produces. For our discussion, the muscles will be grouped according to their primary function, but many of these muscles perform more than one motion.

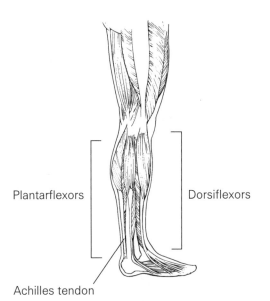

Plantarflexors

Dorsiflexors

Achilles tendon

5.12. The muscles responsible for pointing the foot, curling the toes, and bringing the foot and toes upward

The *plantarflexors* originate at the back of the tibia and fibula and attach to the heel bone (*calcaneus*) via the Achilles tendon (see Figure 5.12). Their function is to point the foot and curl the toes.

The *dorsiflexors* originate at the front of the tibia and fibula and attach to the top of the foot (see Figure 5.12). Their function is to bring the foot and toes upward. This muscle is important because it slows your foot down when you walk. Without this muscle, your foot would flop onto the floor like a clown in oversized shoes. Weakness in this muscle is one of the causes of shin splints (though tight plantarflexors are another predisposing factor).

The *invertors* begin at the front and back of the tibia and fibula and attach to the top and bottom of the inside edge of the foot. Their function is to invert or bring the inside edge of the foot upward. If you are a heavy pronator (flat-footed), it is important for you to strengthen these muscles to maintain the integrity of your arch. It is also highly recommended that you wear orthotics, especially when playing sports (see the "Orthotics" tip in this chapter).

The *evertors* originate at the front and back of the fibula and attach to the bottom and outside of the foot. The function of the evertors is to evert or bring the outside edge of the foot upward. These are the muscles that get weak and stretched out when you sprain your ankle, which then predisposes you to multiple ankle sprains. If you fit this profile, pay special attention to the evertor exercise in the next chapter.

ACHILLES TENDONITIS

Tightness in your plantarflexors predisposes an individual to many foot problems, such as Achilles tendonitis and plantar fascitis. Wearing high-heeled shoes on a daily basis can permanently shorten the Achilles tendon. Also, chronic tendonitis during your 20s and 30s can lead to a full Achilles tendon rupture in your 40s and 50s. When this happens, the only option is surgery, which entails a grueling year of rehabilitation. So always maintain good flexibility in this muscle group. Chapter 10 contains a program for improving calf flexibility.

Your Notes:

Chapter 6

The Lower Extremity Solution

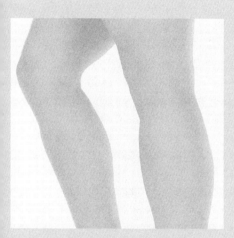

This section addresses strength and alignment issues raised in Chapter 5. That does not mean you should forget everything you learned in the Low Back Solution. We are developing a program for lifelong fitness. You should have already begun integrating the abdominal exercises from Chapter 4 into your everyday life and noticing changes in your alignment and movement pattern. I also recommend that you begin reading Chapter 13, "Choosing *Peak Performance Fitness* for Life," so you can begin to develop your *Peak Performance Fitness* Action Plan.

As discussed in the previous chapter, one of the primary reasons people have lower extremity problems is because of poor alignment, which is often the result of a muscle imbalance. So it is vital throughout the workout that you maintain your alignment as indicated in the photographs and stay activated through your abdominals.

Exercise Overview

There are six exercises in the Lower Extremity Solution program. Three are for the legs and three are for the feet. You may find that you cannot execute many of the exercises correctly, even without a weight. That is okay. It just means you have some long-standing alignment issues that will take some time to work out. Stay true to your

SOCKS

Most people do not give enough thought to the type of sock they wear. A sock not only acts as a barrier between your foot and the shoe, but it also acts as a shock absorber. For this reason, it is vital that the sock fit your foot properly and not slip.

The only kind of socks I ever wear are Thorlos. I discovered them about 6 years ago and have not worn anything else since. Thorlo has a full line of sport-specific socks, but I wear their running and hiking socks all the time, no matter what I'm doing. Why are Thorlos so great? They fit your feet perfectly, the specially reinforced bottoms cushion your foot, and they are so well constructed they last forever.

For ordering information, see Appendix D.

form and within 2 to 3 weeks you will be able to execute the movements for 15 repetitions in good form. The worst thing you could do would be to add weight before you have perfected your form.

The program begins with the straight leg raise, which addresses leg and abdominal muscle endurance. The second exercise, the side-lying leg lift is designed to strengthen and stretch out weak hip abductors. One of the reasons many runners develop a tight iliotibial band (a fibrous structure that extends from your hip to your shin) is because their hip abductors are weak, and the iliotibial band must take up the slack. As a result, it tightens. This can lead to a whole host of problems, such as patellofemoral pain, bursitis of the hip, patella subluxation, and low back pain. It is very easy to cheat on this exercise and use your hip flexors. To prevent this, be exceptionally strict with your form.

The third exercise for the legs is the wall sit. This exercise has been around for years. Wrestlers, martial artists, and soccer players use it. It is primarily intended for quadricep strengthening, but we are going to take it a step further by working on your upper body alignment. We worked on your head, neck, and shoulder alignment in the abdominal section, with you lying on your back. The next step is to remove the support of the floor and bring you into a standing position supported by the wall. Your goal is to eventually be able to maintain good alignment without any external support. It will be a step-by-step process. Please do not get frustrated if you are unable to move beyond the Level 1 wall sit immediately. Remember, if it was easy, everyone would have excellent posture.

The foot section includes exercises to address chronic ankle sprains, shin splints, and pronated feet. Weight guidelines are the same as those for the leg exercises. You need to wear shoes for the first two foot exercises, and as with the abdominal exercises in the Low Back Solution, you must exercise with your midsection visible at all times so you can check your posture. See "What to Wear" in Chapter 4 for more about this.

Equipment Checklist

- A long mirror on its side on the floor so you can watch your form.

- A towel to lie on.

- Adjustable ankle weights.

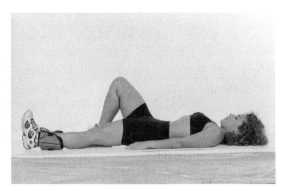

Straight leg raise—Start position

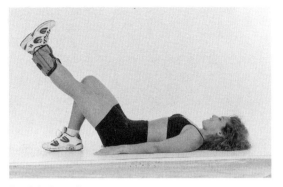

Straight leg raise

Lower Extremity Solution Exercise 1

Straight Leg Raise

1. Place the weight around your ankle.

    The following is a general guide for the first few times you try the exercise:

    Beginner—no weight

    Intermediate—2 pounds

    Master—5 pounds

    Your goal is not to increase the weight you lift, but to perfect your form.

2. Lie on your back with your left leg extended and the right knee bent. Activate your core and keep it activated during the entire exercise while you relax the shoulders and back of the neck onto the floor.

3. Exhale and lift the left leg off the floor, keeping the knee straight. Lift the leg until the knees are even.

4. Inhale and slowly lower the leg to the floor while keeping your navel in and your low back pressed into the floor. Rest 5 seconds. Repeat the above move five times. Based upon your ability to maintain your form during this move, adjust the weight.

Reduce the weight (or remove it) if you are unable to maintain your form, and add additional weight if the exercise seems too easy and you are maintaining perfect form.

5. Repeat the movement ten to fifteen times without stopping. Only the heel should touch the floor. Rest 15 seconds, then repeat the straight leg raise for 2 more sets of 15 repetitions. Repeat the exercise with the right leg.

6. Your ultimate goal is to be able to perform 3 sets of 15 repetitions using a weight that is 10 percent of your body weight.

Check to Make Sure:

■ Foot and knee are facing the ceiling.

■ Low back is anchored to the floor throughout as you lift and lower each leg.

■ Chest is open and backs of shoulders are relaxed onto the floor.

You Should Feel Work Going on In:

■ The front of your thigh and hip.

■ Abdominals.

If you feel work anywhere else, check your form.

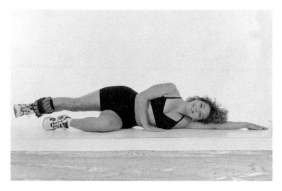

Sidelying leg lift—Start position

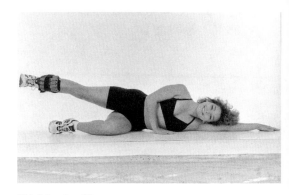

Sidelying leg lift

Lower Extremity Solution Exercise 2

Sidelying Leg Lift

1. Keep the ankle weight on (see Exercise 1 for weight guidelines) and lie on your side facing the mirror. Your alignment should be as follows:

   ■ Hips stacked on top of each other.

   ■ Ear, shoulder, hip, knee, and ankle in one straight line.

2. While lying on your side, bend both knees upward toward your stomach.

3. Straighten the top leg, so that it is again aligned with the rest of your body.

4. Relax your head onto your arm.

5. Exhale and pull in your navel, and lift the top leg while keeping your navel in. Your leg should only be as high as pictured.

6. Inhale and return the leg to the original position. Repeat five times, then adjust the weight up or down depending on how well you maintained your form and how easy the exercise was. Repeat the above movement for 15 repetitions without resting. Rest 15 seconds, then repeat for 2 more sets of 15 repetitions. Repeat the exercise using the other leg.

7. Your ultimate goal is to be able to perform 3 sets of 15 repetitions using a weight that is 10 percent of your body weight.

Check to Make Sure:

■ Your hips are not rolling backward or forward.

■ The knee is straight at the top of the movement. (Use the mirror. Do not look down to check your leg, as this alters your alignment.)

■ Abdominals are activated throughout the exercise. (Use your breathing to help you.)

You Should Feel Work Going on In:

■ The backside of the top hip into the buttock.

■ Abdominals.

If you feel work anywhere else, then check your alignment and relax that area.

Lower Extremity Solution Exercise 3

Level 1: Basic Wall Sit

1. Position the mirror so you can see yourself from the side.

2. Stand 6 inches away from the wall, lean back against the wall, and walk your feet out until both your hips and knees are at an angle slightly above 90 degrees.

3. The following parts of your body should be flush against the wall:

   ■ Low back

   ■ Both shoulder blades

   ■ Back of shoulders

   ■ Base of skull

4. Stay in this position for the allotted amount of time based upon your skill level:

   Beginner—30 seconds

   Intermediate—60 seconds

   Master—2 minutes

5. Activate your core while keeping the body parts that are listed in step 3 flush against the wall.

6. After your time has elapsed, come out of the position, rest for 15 seconds, and repeat the exercise two more times.

Check to Make Sure:

■ The body parts listed in step 3 remain flush against the wall.

■ Chin is tucked in.

■ No hands on thighs—that is called "cheating."

You Should Feel Work Going on In:

■ Quadriceps.

■ Abdominals.

■ Mild stretching in portions of upper back and chest.

Note: *If you feel knee pain when performing this exercise, compare your knee alignment to the picture and adjust accordingly. If you continue to have knee pain, discontinue this exercise until you can perform Lower Extremity Exercise 1 with 10 percent of your body weight.*

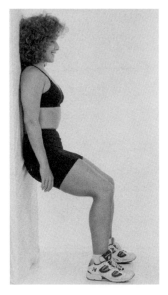

Level 1: Basic wall sit

Level 2: Wall Sit with External Rotation of the Arms

1. Assume the wall-sitting position described in Level 1, then reach forward with your arms and bring them straight back so that your elbows are touching the wall.

2. Keep your back and head anchored to the wall while rotating both forearms up so that the backs of your hands are touching the wall.

3. If your elbows or knuckles do not touch the wall, keep performing the exercise. In time they will.

4. Hold this position for the allotted time depending on your experience level:

   Beginner—30 seconds

   Intermediate—60 seconds

   Master—2 minutes

5. After your time has elapsed, come out of the position, rest for 15 seconds, and repeat the exercise two more times.

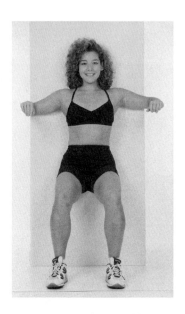

Level 2: Wall sit–Start position

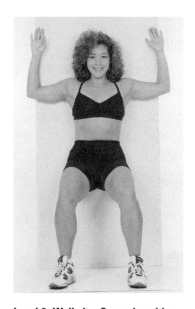

Level 2: Wall sit—Second position

Level 3: Wall Sit with External Rotation Slides

1. Assume the sitting, arms-out position described in Level 2. However, once you can touch your elbows and knuckles to the wall, slide your arms up and down the wall while keeping your head and back anchored to the wall. Slide your arms only as high as you can while keeping your body anchored. This too will eventually improve with time. Repeat the up-and-down sliding motion as many times as you can for the allotted time period for your level. Rest for 15 seconds and repeat the exercise two more times.

Note: If you have pain in your shoulder(s) while performing the arm motion, check your alignment. If pain persists, consult your orthopedist because you may have a shoulder problem, and this upward movement will make it worse.

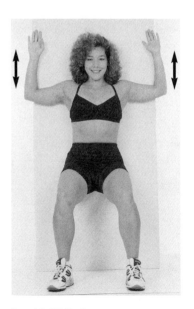

Level 3: Wall sit

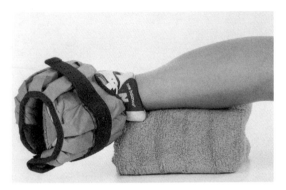

Ankle eversion—Start position

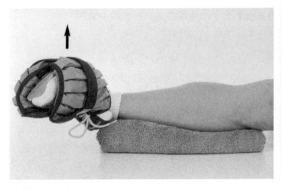

Ankle eversion

Lower Extremity Solution Exercise 4

Ankle Eversion

1. With your shoe on, strap the ankle weight to your forefoot (see Lower Extremity Solution Exercise 1 for weight guideline).

2. Lie on your side in good alignment and place the top leg on a folded towel.

3. Lift the side of your foot up toward the ceiling for 3 sets of 15 repetitions. Control the motion both up and down. Letting the ankle flop down could cause injury and defeats the purpose of the exercise. Rest for 15 seconds between each set.

4. Repeat the exercise with the other foot.

Check to Make Sure:

■ You have full ankle range motion during exercise.

You Should Feel Work Going on In:

■ Outside of lower leg.

Lower Extremity Solution Exercise 5

Ankle Dorsiflexion

1. With the ankle weight on your forefoot, sit on a high table, chair, or kitchen counter, so that your feet cannot touch the ground.

2. While maintaining good alignment, lift your forefoot toward your shin for 3 sets of 15 repetitions. Again, control the motion both up and down. Rest for 15 seconds between each set.

Check to Make Sure:

■ You are sitting up straight with navel in.

■ You have full ankle range motion during exercise.

You Should Feel Work Going on In:

■ Front of shin.

■ Achilles tendon.

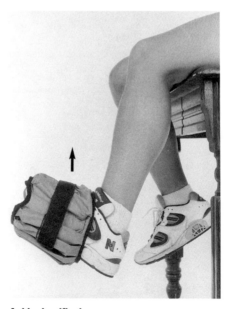

Ankle dorsiflexion

Lower Extremity Solution Exercise 6

Towel Grabs

1. Remove the weight from your forefoot; sit in a chair with a towel under your bare feet.

2. Grab the towel with your toes one hundred times.

Check to Make Sure:

- You are sitting in good alignment.

- The toes are curling completely under for each repetition.

You Should Feel Work Going on In:

- This is not an exercise that goes for the "burn." That is all right; it is still effective.

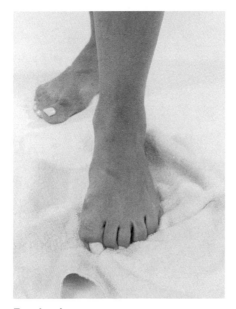

Towel grabs

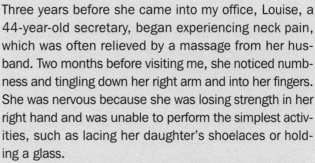

Chapter 7

Why Biceps Curls Are a Waste of Your Time

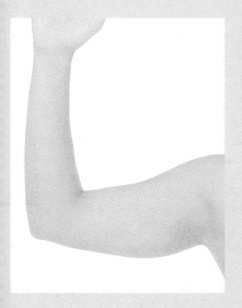

Three years before she came into my office, Louise, a 44-year-old secretary, began experiencing neck pain, which was often relieved by a massage from her husband. Two months before visiting me, she noticed numbness and tingling down her right arm and into her fingers. She was nervous because she was losing strength in her right hand and was unable to perform the simplest activities, such as lacing her daughter's shoelaces or holding a glass.

Louise worked from 9 a.m. to 5 p.m. everyday. Most of her time was spent typing on the computer with the telephone cradled on her shoulder. Three days a week during her lunch break she exercised at the company's health club. Her routine consisted of walking on the treadmill for 30 minutes and a 30-minute weight training routine that focused on her chest and arms.

What was Louise's diagnosis? She had moderate neck, chest, and shoulder muscle tightness, complicated by a herniated disc. As discussed in Chapter 3, good alignment puts your body in its optimal functioning position. Each bone, ligament, and muscle has an optimal resting position and movement pattern. If this pattern is altered, then that bone, ligament, or muscle no longer operates efficiently, predisposing it and surrounding structures to premature breakdown. In the upper body, this breakdown can manifest itself in the following ailments:

- Headaches

- Neck spasms

- Herniated discs

- Rotator cuff impingement (shoulder pain)

- Rotator cuff tear

- Cervical osteoarthritis

- Tennis elbow

- TMJ (temporamandibular jaw) problems

In Louise's case, her sedentary job was compromising her posture and her exercise routine was contributing to her poor alignment. Because of her slumped sitting posture, Louise's upper back muscles had become over-stretched and weak. She also sat with her head hanging out in front of her body. The average weight of the human head is 10 pounds when properly aligned over the spinal column.

WHAT IS BURSITIS?

A **bursa** is a fluid sac whose job is to prevent friction. Bursas are found all over your body. They are in your knees, hips, shoulders…everywhere. When a bursa is traumatized, it becomes inflamed and swells up. This is called **bursitis.** The best way to treat bursitis is to remove the irritant. In many cases, this means temporarily stopping the activity or movement pattern that is producing the trauma.

WHERE DO YOU HOLD YOUR STRESS?

There are two times that people recruit their **upper trapezius muscle,** located on the upper back, when they should not. The first is to compensate for weakness during exercises by shrugging (lifting their shoulders). Do not shrug unless you want a wrestler's neck. Second, people scrunch up when they are stressed. Relax this muscle when you exercise and when you are tense. A good way to prevent this stress-holding pattern is to do 10 shoulder rolls every 2 hours when you are at work or in a stressful situation.

Because your bones are designed to be weight-bearing structures, this generally works out fine. If your head is positioned a few inches forward, however, the force on your vertebrae changes, causing your muscles to contract excessively to hold your head in place. Holding your head in this forward position for an extended period of time causes a nice neck spasm. If this position is maintained over time, your muscles will shorten and reversal of this condition becomes increasingly difficult. Continued over a period of years, this condition will likely lead to a herniated disc and arthritis of your cervical spine, and eventually your bones will fuse in this position.

When it came to her exercise routine, Louise made the mistake most people make. She exercised what she saw in the mirror, her chest and arms, when in fact she should have been strengthening her upper and lower back muscles. When you exercise the large muscles of the upper and lower back, you recruit the arm muscles, thereby strengthening them. This is why biceps curls are a waste of your time. Take the time that you would spend exercising your biceps and focus on strengthening your upper back muscles. Also, since her chest muscles were tight from her sitting posture, they were the last thing she needed to work on.

In this chapter, we examine the common causes of neck and shoulder pain. Both problems are on a continuum and are easily reversed if they are recognized early enough. Most neck problems (including herniated discs) are the result of uneven weight-bearing through the spine, and all shoulder injuries are the result of compromised space in the shoulder joint, and so the key to prevention is maintenance of healthy alignment in both joints. This healthy alignment is achieved by good posture, which is maintained by strong, endurance-driven upper back and rotator cuff muscles. Chapter 8, "The Upper Extremity Solution," is the comprehensive program that will help you achieve this.

Louise's Problem

On Louise's first visit, I explained that her condition was very treatable and that we needed to improve her posture since this was the primary cause of her herniated disc. As we saw in Chapter 3, disc herniations usually occur as a result of uneven weight-bearing through the vertebrae. This causes the disks, which are located between the vertebrae, to get pushed out of alignment. In many cases, the disc presses on a nerve, and you usually will not get symptoms until that occurs. The symptom is typically a tingling or weakness radiating down the arm. The type of nerve that the disc is pressing on will determine the location of the

OCCIPIVOT

The occipivot is a device that I ask many of my neck patients to purchase for home use. It enables them to apply trigger-point therapy to their neck muscles. A trigger point is a point of hyperirritability in a muscle. This can develop whenever a muscle is held in an unnatural position for a prolonged period of time. Sitting hunched over the computer or frequently cradling the telephone on your shoulder are perfect ways to develop a trigger point in your neck. In fact, the neck is one of the more common areas where individuals develop trigger points. Individuals who carry tension in this area experience headaches, temporamandibular jaw (TMJ) dysfunction, and a feeling of compression in the neck region.

The fingerlike projections of the occipivot apply gentle pressure to the muscles at the base of your skull. (The area where your skull meets your neck is referred to as your **occiput**.) This pressure interrupts the excess neural activity in the muscle and forces it to relax. It also increases the blood flow to the area, which brings oxygen and nutrients to the tissue, thereby removing the pain-inducing metabolic wastes.

The occipivot is not the total answer to neck pain, but it can be part of the solution. You still need to determine why your neck hurts and adjust your alignment appropriately.

Precaution: Do not use the occipivot if you have rheumatoid arthritis or Down's syndrome or have suffered neck trauma. These conditions can compromise the integrity of your neck ligaments, in which case the muscle spasm may be vital for maintaining your neck stability. For ordering information, see Appendix D.

symptoms and what muscles are affected. Disc herniations can range from a faint tingling sensation in the shoulder area to a complete loss of muscle strength and function in the affected upper extremity, which was beginning to happen to Louise. Depending upon the severity and duration of the symptoms, the loss can be temporary or permanent. Disc herniations can occur anywhere in the spine. Prevention of a herniated disc requires the even distribution of weight through your vertebrae. This is accomplished by—you guessed it—good alignment.

The Second Half of Louise's Problem

The herniated disc was only half of Louise's problem. She also had moderate neck, chest, and shoulder fascial tightness. As discussed in Chapter 3, fascia is a tough fibrous connective tissue that surrounds your muscles, organs, and nerves. Fascia is a three-dimensional weblike structure that holds everything in place.

When fascia tightens in the cervical region, many structures are affected. Exiting out between your cervical vertebrae and passing beneath your collarbone are numerous nerves and blood vessels. If the fascia and muscles in this area get too tight, you will not only experience neck spasm pain, but you are likely to develop symptoms down your arm, such as weakness, coldness, or loss of sensation.

This is important to remember because the neck and shoulders are one of the primary areas where many of us hold our stress. This tension, often combined with poor sitting alignment for 8 hours a day at work, can set an individual up for a lifetime of pain. Rather than medication, persons with these symptoms should learn to sit up straight, strengthen their muscles to maintain proper alignment, and develop outlets for their stress, such as regular exercise.

Wham, Wham, Wham!

Malalignment and poor upper back muscle endurance are not only the culprits in neck pain, but in shoulder pain as well. Jonathan, a 24-year-old tennis player, had been experiencing shoulder pain for 5 months. Jonathan only experienced pain when he raised his arm above his shoulders (above 90 degrees) and when he tried to serve.

Jonathan's complaints point to a very common shoulder issue. There is a finite amount of space available in the shoulder joint, and the joint is crowded with many structures, including a bursa and one of the rotator cuff tendons (*supraspinatus*). It's like trying to navigate your grocery cart down a crowded supermarket aisle. If everyone moves in a predictable pattern, then everyone gets where they need to go. However, if one person deviates or stops short, or if a display stand falls, then everyone backs up and

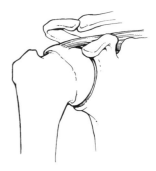

7.1. A healthy shoulder

problems occur. This is what happens every time you lift your arm. Normally, your shoulder joint bones move in such a way so as not to collide with the surrounding structures. When a collision occurs, you have pain. The more frequent the collisions, the more serious the shoulder problem.

Upon evaluation, it was determined that although Jonathan's rotator cuff and upper back muscles were strong, they lacked the endurance and timing necessary for a sport such as tennis. Jonathan would start his game feeling strong, but after 30 minutes of play his form would begin to suffer as his muscles tired. Jonathan also stood with both shoulders rounded forward. This poor shoulder alignment further decreased his shoulder joint space, making collisions in the joint more likely.

Most shoulder problems exist on a continuum from problems that can be reversed with exercise to problems requiring surgery. Jonathan's problem was that he had a rotator cuff impingement that was on the mild end of the continuum (see Figure 7.2).

A rotator cuff impingement is when the rotator cuff tendon hits one of the shoulder joint bones every time the arm is lifted higher than 90 degrees. Symptoms of an impingement are shoulder pain whenever the arm is lifted higher than 90 degrees and pain at the end range of motions. For example, scratching your back or reaching overhead are typical activities that would elicit rotator cuff impingement pain. Impingement can be the result of bad posture, weak muscles, insufficient muscle endurance, and/or poor technique.

Jonathan's problem was a simple one that we corrected with rest and by using the exercises in the next chapter for strengthening the

upper back and rotator cuff muscles. After only 6 weeks of the Upper Extremity Solution, Jonathan was free of pain. He continued to do the exercises to prevent future shoulder problems and because he liked the way they made his body look.

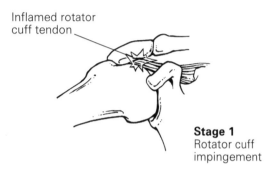

Inflamed rotator cuff tendon

Stage 1
Rotator cuff impingement

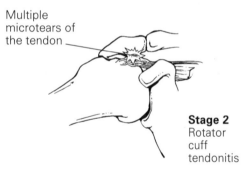

Multiple microtears of the tendon

Stage 2
Rotator cuff tendonitis

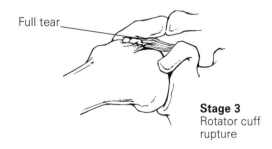

Full tear

Stage 3
Rotator cuff rupture

7.2. The three stages of shoulder problems

ONE SHOULDER EXERCISE IS ENOUGH

People tend to focus a lot of their strength training on their **deltoids**, since they are so visible in the mirror. If your deltoids are too strong and your rotator cuff muscles are weak, then you will be prone to impingement. Most of your upper body strength training should focus on your upper back muscles, such as your **rhomboids, middle trapezius, latissimus dorsi,** and **rotator cuff muscles.** Since the rotator cuff needs to balance the deltoids, your weight and repetitions for both should match. If you are doing 45 repetitions of a 5-pound deltoid raise to the front, then you should be able to perform the "sidelying external rotation" exercise in the Upper Extremity Solution for 45 repetitions with a 5-pound weight also.

However, if Jonathan had not addressed his shoulder problem, it would have developed into rotator cuff tendonitis (see Figure 7.2). Tendonitis results when the impingement becomes a regular problem, and there are multiple microtears of the supraspinatus tendon. Symptoms of rotator cuff tendonitis are moderate pain and weakness on any overhead motion. Opening an umbrella or putting on a jacket are typical activities that would irritate a shoulder with tendonitis. When this irritation goes on for years, a full rotator cuff tear occurs (see Figure 7.2). Every time you experience tendonitis, there is a breaking down and a rebuilding of the tendon. However, the tendon that is rebuilt is never as strong as the original. This means that after many years of chronic tendonitis, you are left with a weakened patchwork tendon that is prone to a full rupture. This is why most rotator cuff tear patients are above the age of 55. Symptoms of a full rotator cuff tear are weakness but no pain on overhead motions. Tendonitis can usually be resolved with exercise and proper alignment. Typically, the only treatment option for a full rotator cuff tear is reconstructive surgery, which can entail 4 to 6 months of painful rehabilitation. Remember, prevention is always the best medicine.

What follows is an in-depth discussion of the upper extremity muscles and tips for maximizing upper extremity performance.

Anatomy Lesson #7:
The Shoulder Complex

The shoulder complex consists of the breast-bone (*sternum*), collarbone (*clavicle*), shoulder blade (*scapula*), and the upper arm bone (*humerus*) (see Figure 7.3).

There are joints between each of these bones. The one that most people have problems with is the connection between the upper arm bone and the shoulder blade, or the *gleno-humeral joint*. This joint is highly mobile, and its purpose is to move your hand and put it in the best position for you to interact with the world. The movements of the shoulder joint are flexion, abduction, and internal and external rotation (see Figure 7.4).

Scapular Stabilizers

There are three main upper back muscles that help stabilize the shoulder blade and ensure that proper shoulder motion is maintained. This is why most of your upper extremity exercises should focus on these and your rotator cuff

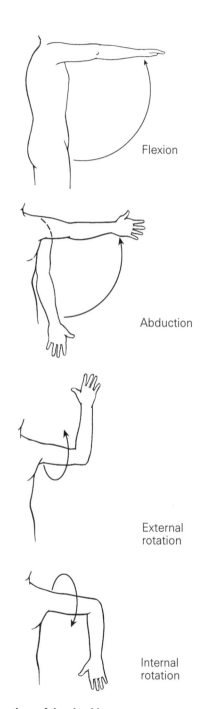

Flexion

Abduction

External rotation

Internal rotation

7.4. The motions of the shoulder

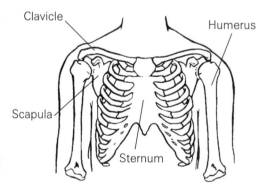

Clavicle

Humerus

Scapula

Sternum

7.3. The shoulder complex

muscles. Having strong upper back muscles will help prevent shoulder problems and improve your posture.

The serratus anterior begins at ribs one through eight and attaches to the inside of the underside of the shoulder blade (see Figure 7.5). The function of the serratus is to hold the shoulder blade against the trunk during arm movements. If you want a lean torso, then you need to work your serratus. The serratus muscle not only affects your arm but your abdominals as well. The serratus attaches to the abdominal fascia, which is one of the two fascial networks responsible for protecting your spine. A strong serratus will slim down the area beneath your armpits.

The rhomboids begin at the last cervical vertebra and the first five thoracic vertebra (T1 to T5) and end at the inside border of the shoulder blade (see Figure 7.6). Their job is to retract the shoulder blade toward the vertebral column. If you are an overhead athlete, it is vital that your rhomboid muscles be strong. If you are unable to retract your shoulder blade, you will pick up the motion at your shoulder and set yourself up for a shoulder problem. This is also a very important postural muscle.

The trapezius muscle originates from the base of the skull to the T12 vertebra and attaches to various areas of the collarbone and shoulder blade (see Figure 7.7). Each section of the trapezius muscle has a specialized function. The upper fibers elevate the shoulder, the middle fibers retract the shoulder blade, and the lower fibers pull the shoulder blade down.

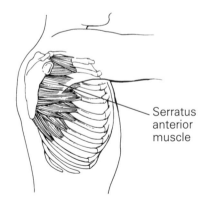

7.5. The muscle responsible for holding the shoulder blade against the trunk during arm movements

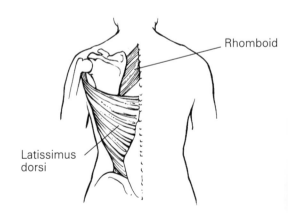

7.6. The muscles responsible for retracting the shoulder blade toward the vertebral column and extending and rotating the upper arm bone

Move That Baby

The following muscles connect the shoulder blade to the upper arm bone. These are the muscles that actually move the upper arm bone.

The deltoid muscle begins at the collarbone and shoulder blade and attaches to the top of the upper arm bone (see Figure 7.7). Its function is to lift the arm to either the front, side, or back.

The latissimus dorsi spans the length of the low back. It originates off various areas of the thoracic spine, hipbone, and ribs. Its final attachment point is on the front of the upper arm bone. This large muscle's function is to extend and rotate the upper arm bone. (See Figure 7.6 to view the latissimus dorsi.) This muscle gives elite swimmers the distinctive V-shape to their backs.

The rotator cuff muscles are a group of four different muscles: the supraspinatus, *subscapularis, teres minor,* and *infraspinatus* (see Figure 7.8). Each one has a specialized function, but in general their role is to rotate the arm and pull the upper arm bone down into the shoulder joint so impingement does not occur. They originate off of different parts of the shoulder blade and all attach to the top of the upper arm bone. Strong rotator cuff muscles with good endurance are one of the primary keys to preventing shoulder problems. Chapter 8 presents a comprehensive exercise program for developing these muscles.

The triceps begin at the back side of the shoulder blade and upper arm bone and attach to the forearm (see Figure 7.8). Their main role is to extend the forearm. Clients often ask what is the best exercise for this muscle so that they can rid themselves of flabby underarms. Again, there is no such thing as a spot reduction exercise. If you tend to deposit fat on the under-

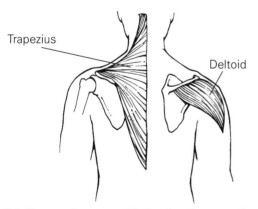

7.7. The muscles responsible for elevating, retracting, and pulling the shoulder blade down as well as lifting the arm

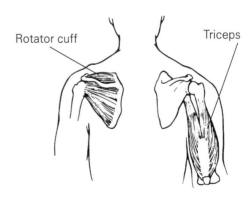

7.8. Rotator cuff and triceps muscles

IMPROVE YOUR CONFIDENCE IN ONE SIMPLE STEP

In most people, the pectoralis major is too tight and contributes to a slumped posture. If your postural evaluation in Chapter 1 revealed that you have rounded shoulders, then you probably have tight pectoralis muscles. This slumped posture predisposes an individual to both neck and shoulder problems. Also, studies have shown that individuals with slumped postures are perceived as being insecure and depressed, while individuals with good posture are perceived as confident and happy. So if you want to look confident, do 10 shoulder rolls and open your chest before any important meeting.

side of your upper arm, the best way to address that area is through a comprehensive cardiovascular and general strengthening program.

The *pectoralis major* originates from different areas of the collarbone and breastbone and attaches to the upper arm bone (see Figure 7.9). The function of this strong muscle is to flex, extend, and rotate the upper arm bone.

The biceps begin at the front tip of shoulder blade and attach to the forearm (see Figure 7.9). Their function is to flex the upper arm bone and also to rotate the forearm. I often see patients who have been diagnosed with biceps tendonitis. Biceps tendonitis as an isolated problem is rare. Because of the way the shoulder functions, biceps tendonitis is typically secondary to a rotator cuff problem. Many researchers believe that biceps tendon soreness is a precursor to impingement. For this reason, it is wisest to spend your time strengthening your upper back and rotator cuff muscles. This is another reason why biceps curls are a waste of time.

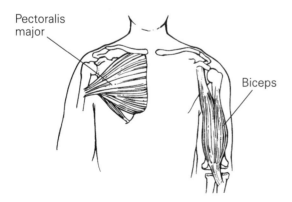

Pectoralis major

Biceps

7.9. Pectoralis major and biceps muscles

Chapter 8

The Upper Extremity Solution

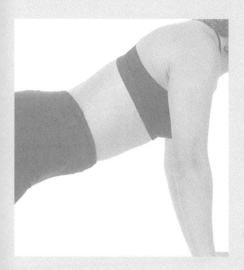

The Upper Extremity Solution consists of four exercises, all designed to improve the strength and endurance of your upper back and rotator cuff muscles. Upper Extremity Exercise 1 addresses the rotator cuff muscles, which move the upper arm bone downward when the arm is lifted. Remember, if the upper arm bone is not depressed in the shoulder joint when the arm is raised, then the rotator cuff will impinge, which can lead to tendonitis and eventually to a complete tear.

In the second exercise you will learn, or relearn, push-ups. Push-ups are great. They are a multijoint exercise—meaning they use several joints and muscles simultaneously, working your chest, upper back, and arms while using your body weight as resistance. All weight-bearing exercises are good for joint and bone nutrition. In sum, push-ups are an efficient, portable exercise that lets you hit many muscles quickly.

For the third exercise, chair dips, you will need a sturdy chair and the mirror. Chair dips are another multijoint exercise, and they are excellent for strengthening and postural alignment if you do them in good form. Initially, you may not be able to keep your back straight throughout the exercise. That is all right. Continue the exercise, but limit the depth of the dip to the point where you can still maintain a straight back. After a couple of weeks, these inflexibilities will work themselves out and you will notice that you can increase your range while maintaining good form.

The final exercise is facedown rows. This exercise is excellent for strengthening your middle trapezius and rhomboids, both of which are very important for maintaining good posture. If you sit in a slumped position all day, these muscles become stretched out and weak and predispose you to numerous neck and shoulder problems.

As with all the exercises in this book, you need to exercise with your torso exposed so you can monitor your posture; see "What to Wear" in Chapter 4 for more on this. Also, as you integrate more exercises into your routine, you may want to begin reading Chapter 13, "Choosing *Peak Performance Fitness* for Life," which will help you integrate the *Peak Performance Fitness* program into your life and guarantee your success.

Equipment Checklist

- A mirror to monitor your form.

- A small towel folded into a compact bundle.

- A sturdy armless chair; a folding chair is fine, so long as it's strong.

- Adjustable weights.

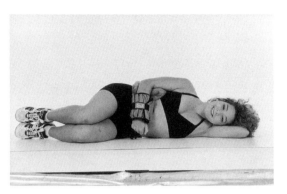

Sidelying external rotation—Start position

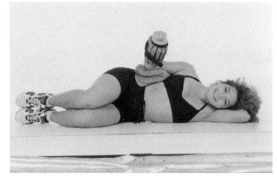

Sidelying external rotation—Second position

Upper Extremity Solution Exercise 1

Sidelying External Rotation

1. Wrap the weight around your right wrist.

   How much weight should you use? Follow this general guide:

   Beginner—no weight

   Intermediate—2 pounds

   Master—5 pounds

2. Lie on your left side facing the mirror with your head resting on your arm or a pillow. Using the mirror, make sure your ear, shoulder, hip, and knee are in a straight line. Then bend your hips and knees to approximately 45 degrees while keeping your upper body aligned.

3. Place the small towel between your right elbow and right ribcage.

4. Bend the right elbow to ninety degrees and rest the arm across the front of your body.

5. Exhale, pull your navel in, and slowly rotate your right forearm upward until the forearm is perpendicular to the floor.

6. Inhale as you return the arm to its resting position.

7. Do 10 to 15 repetitions without stopping. Rest for 15 seconds and repeat the exercise again for 2 more sets of 10 to 15 repetitions. Repeat the exercise on the left arm.

8. Your ultimate goal is to be able to perform the exercise for 3 sets of 15 repetitions using a weight that is 5 to 7 percent of your body weight. So if you are 130 pounds, eventually you should be lifting 6.5 to 9 pounds.

Check to Make Sure:

- Your shoulders are relaxed away from your ears.

- Your elbow is tucked into your ribcage.

You Should Feel Work Going on In:

- Back of upper arm.

- Abdominals.

Upper Extremity Solution Exercise 2

Level 1: Wall Push-Ups

1. Stand approximately 2 feet away from the wall with the mirror facing your side.

2. Place your hands shoulder-width apart on the wall, arms straight. Your hands should be directly in front of your shoulders.

3. Look at the wall, inhale, and bend your elbows until your face is 2 inches away from the wall.

4. Exhale, pull your navel in, straighten your elbows, and imagine that you are pushing the wall away.

5. Do 5 to 10 repetitions. Rest for 15 seconds, then repeat the exercise for 2 more sets of 5 to 10 repetitions.

6. Once you can perform 3 sets of 10 in good form, move on to Level 2.

Check to Make Sure:

■ Your hands are directly in front of your shoulders.

■ Your entire back is flat throughout the exercise. Use the mirror for monitoring.

■ Your elbows are bending back toward you.

■ There is even weight distribution between your arms.

■ Your elbows are not locked at any time. This will injure your elbows.

You Should Feel Work Going on In:

■ Triceps (back of upper arm).

■ Abdominals.

■ Pectoralis major (chest).

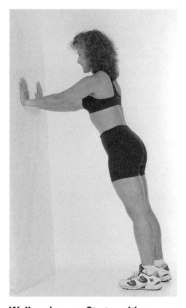

Wall push-ups—Start position

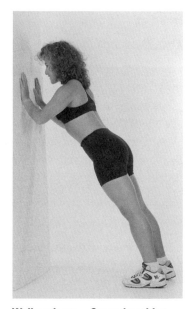

Wall push-ups—Second position

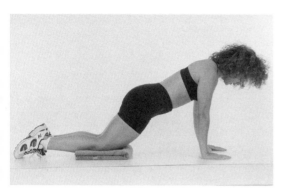

Bent knee push-ups—Start position

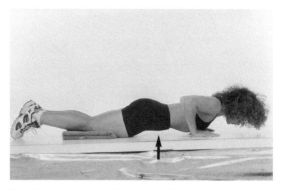

Bent knee push-ups—Second position

Level 2: Bent Knee Push-Ups

1. Position the mirror on the floor next to you.

2. Assume a quadruped position.

3. Walk your hands forward approximately 6 inches and flatten your low back by tucking your buttocks under.

4. Inhale and bend your elbows (while keeping your back straight) until your chest (not your head) is about 4 inches from the floor.

5. Exhale, pull your navel in, and push the floor away until your elbows are straight. Do not lock or pop your elbows while in the up position. This can injure your elbows.

6. Do 5 to 10 repetitions. Rest 15 seconds, then repeat the exercise for 2 more sets of 5 to 10 repetitions.

7. Once you can perform 3 sets of 10 repetitions in perfect form, progress to Level 3.

Check to Make Sure:

- Shoulders are relaxed and neck is long.

- Head, shoulders, hip, and knee are in one straight line. No droopy heads!

- Elbows are bending back toward the body.

You Should Feel Work Going on In:

- Anterior deltoids (front of shoulder).

- Triceps.

- Abdominals.

- Pectorals.

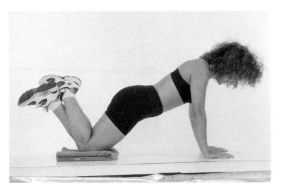

Bent knee push-ups with feet lifted—Start position

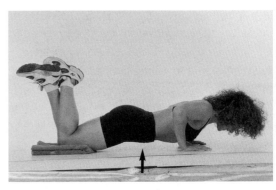

Bent knee push-ups with feet lifted—Second position

Level 3: Bent Knee Push-Ups with Feet Lifted

1. Repeat Level 2 steps 1 to 3, then lift your feet off the floor and cross your ankles.

2. Inhale and bend your elbows until your chest is about 4 inches from the floor.

3. Exhale, pull your navel in, and push the floor away until your elbows are almost straight.

4. Do 5 to 10 repetitions. Rest 15 seconds, then repeat the exercise for 2 more sets of 5 to 10 repetitions.

5. Once you can perform 3 sets of 10 repetitions in perfect form, progress to Level 4.

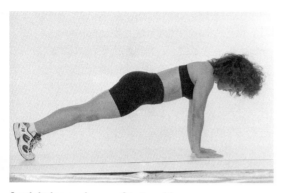

Straight leg push-ups—Start position

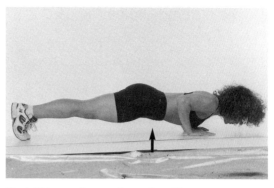

Straight leg push-ups—Second position

Level 4: Straight Leg Push-Ups

1. Repeat Level 2 steps 1 to 3. Walk your right foot, and then your left foot, backward until your knees are straight.

2. Inhale and bend your elbows until your chest is about 4 inches from the floor.

3. Exhale, pull your navel in, and push the floor away until your elbows are almost straight. Again, do not pop or lock your elbows in the up position.

4. Do 5 to 10 repetitions. Rest 15 seconds, then repeat the exercise for 2 more sets of 5 to 10 repetitions.

5. Your ultimate goal for this exercise is to be able to execute 3 sets of 15 repetitions in good form. Once you are able to do this, keep increasing the number of repetitions until you are doing 60 push-ups each session.

Upper Extremity Solution Exercise 3

Level 1: Chair Dips with Knees Flexed

1. Place the mirror next to the chair.

2. Sit on the edge of the chair with your hands grasping either side of the chair seat, knuckles facing outward. Bend your hips and knees to 90 degrees with your feet wide apart.

3. Keep your chest open, neck long, navel in, and move your buttocks completely off the front of the chair.

4. Inhale and then bend your elbows. Ultimately, your goal is to bend your elbows to almost 90 degrees in good form. For now, begin with small arcs of movement through the elbow and progress until you can bend your elbows to 90 degrees on the downward motion while maintaining a straight back. Try to duplicate the shoulder, hip, and knee alignment in the picture.

5. Exhale, pull your navel in, and push up from the chair (as if pushing the chair away) until your elbows are almost straight.

6. Do 5 to 10 repetitions without stopping. Rest 15 seconds and then repeat the exercise for 2 more sets of 5 to 10 repetitions.

7. When you can perform 3 sets of 10 repetitions in good form with the elbows bent to 90 degrees, progress to Level 2.

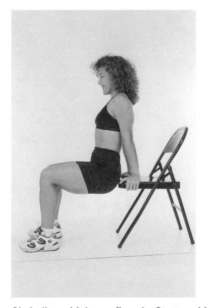

Chair dips with knees flexed—Start position

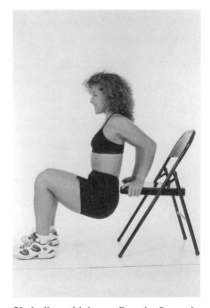

Chair dips with knees flexed—Second position

Check to Make Sure:

- Your neck is long, chest is open, and navel is in.

- Your elbows are bending backward, not out to the side.

- Your buttocks and low back are brushing up against the chair throughout the exercise.

- You do not go below 90 degrees of elbow flexion.

- You are using the mirror to check your alignment.

You Should Feel Work Going on In:

- Triceps.

- Chest.

- Abdominals.

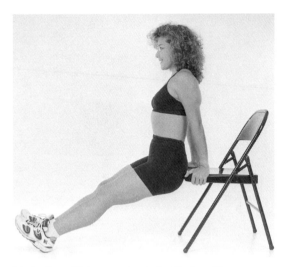

Chair dips with knees extended—Start position

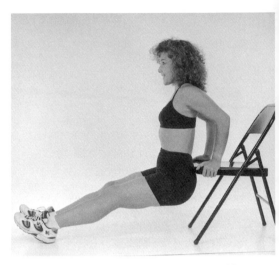

Chair dips with knees extended—Second position

Level 2: Chair Dips with Knees Extended

1. Repeat Level 1 steps 1 to 6, except instead of flexing your knees, extend them straight, with heels resting on floor.

2. Your goal is to be able to perform 3 sets of 15 repetitions in perfect form. Use the mirror to check your form.

Check to Make Sure:

- Your neck is long, chest is open, and navel is in throughout the exercise.

- Your elbows are bending backward.

- Your buttocks and lower back are brushing up against the chair throughout the exercise. Your back should be completely straight.

You Should Feel Work Going on In:

- Triceps.

- Chest.

Upper Extremity Solution Exercise 4

Facedown Rows

1. Wrap the weight around your right wrist.

   The following is a general weight guide:

   Beginner—no weight

   Intermediate—2 pounds

   Master—5 pounds

2. Bend over your kitchen table or desk so that your right arm is hanging off the side. Rest your forehead on a small towel so you have enough room to breathe.

3. During the exercise your neck and shoulders should remain relaxed. Exhale, bend your elbow to 90 degrees, and lift the elbow toward the ceiling while squeezing the right shoulder blade back.

4. Inhale and slowly lower the arm back down toward the floor. Do 10 to 15 repetitions without stopping. Rest 15 seconds and repeat the exercise for 2 more sets of 10 to 15 repetitions. Repeat the exercise on the left arm.

5. Your ultimate goal is to be able to perform 3 sets of 15 repetitions using a weight that equals 5 percent of your body weight.

Check to Make Sure That:

- Your neck and shoulders are relaxed.

- Your forehead is resting on a small towel roll.

- You are pinching your shoulder blade back.

You Should Feel Work Going on In:

- Triceps (back of arm).

- Middle trapezius and rhomboids (the muscles between your shoulder blade and spine).

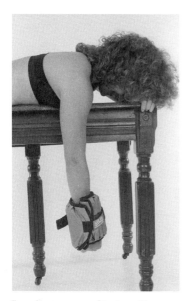

Facedown rows—Start position

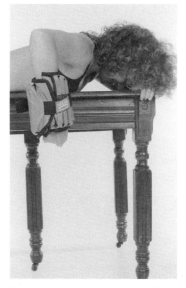

Facedown rows—Second position

Your Notes:

Chapter 9

Why You Should Never Stretch Before Exercising...

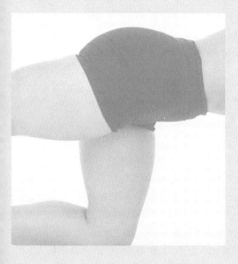

Here is a quick quiz: Which one of the following individuals needs flexibility training the most?

A. Olympic gymnast

B. 55-year-old lawyer

C. You

D. All of the above

You guessed it! The correct answer is D. Every individual listed needs flexibility training. Every muscle has an optimal length or position. If the muscle is too long or too short, then it does not operate efficiently, and it affects the efficiency of surrounding muscles. The perfect example was David, a 55-year-old lawyer who sat at his desk 10 hours a day in a slumped posture. His shoulders were rounded forward with a huge upper back kyphosis (a backward curve of the spine), and his head jutted forward in front of his body. An analysis of his muscles revealed that his chest muscles were short and tight, while his upper back muscles were stretched out and weak. This inflexibility was pulling his neck, jaw, and shoulders into an unnatural position. His neck muscles were going into spasm because they were working overtime to hold his head over his body, which was also affecting the alignment of his jaw. David was having severe jaw pain with radiating headaches and intermittent jaw "clicking." It was the jaw pain that brought David to see me. After 12 weeks on the *Peak Performance Fitness* exercise program, including the flexibility and breathing exercises here and in the next chapter, David was free of pain and there were visible improvements in his posture. The jaw pain also caused David to review his schedule and make a concerted effort to include exercise on a daily basis.

In this and the next chapter we will develop a flexibility training program, while being mindful of all that we have learned to this point about proper alignment.

…Or Why You Don't Store Rubber Bands in the Freezer

Flexibility is the range of motion available at a joint (where bone meets bone), and the flexibility available is dependent upon four factors: bone structure of the joint, ligaments, length of the muscles and tendons surrounding the joint, and neuromuscular responses. Of the four factors, we can only effect change in two: in the muscles and tendons and in the neuromuscular responses. The best way of increasing the flexibility of the muscle and tendon is by heating them up (through exercise) and then holding them in a lengthened position for a minimum of 60 seconds. Your muscles and tendons contain an elastic component (like a rubber band). Like any elastic substance, they are most pliable when they are warm. If you try to stretch them when they are cold, you run the risk of tearing a muscle or tendon. This is why you should *never* stretch before you exercise.

A neuromuscular response is the order in which and the magnitude to which your body decides to use a muscle for a particular movement. For example, in Chapter 5 we learned that at the knee there is a constant tug-of-war between the muscles for control of your kneecap. If both medial and lateral thigh muscles "turn on" simultaneously and with equal magnitude, the kneecap will track properly. However, if one muscle is delayed or unable to match the power of the other, the kneecap tracks incorrectly and knee pain ensues. Proper kneecap tracking is an example of when order and magnitude must be equal. Lifting your arm is another example. The rotator cuff muscles must be able to match the timing and magnitude of the deltoid muscles and pull the upper arm bone downward in the shoulder joint. Otherwise, the upper arm bone pushes the rotator cuff tendon into the shoulder joint and shoulder pain occurs. However, there are cases in the body where it is vital that one muscle's activation precedes that of other muscles. In Chapter 3 we learned that a delayed response of the transversus abdominis muscle is the reason many back patients continue to reinjure themselves. Transversus abdominis' activation must precede that of all other muscles because this muscle's job is to corset or protect the spine before movement occurs.

Why Flexibility Training Is Important

The exercise program you have built to this point, which is designed to improve your alignment, improves the neuromuscular response of your muscles and also increases your dynamic flexibility. There are two different types of flexibility, dynamic and static. Dynamic flexibility is the ability of your muscles to lengthen and shorten efficiently through large ranges of motion when you are moving. The ability of a dancer to kick her leg overhead is an example of someone who has exceptional dynamic flexibility in her legs. Most of us do not require this extreme range in our everyday lives. However, good dynamic flexibility does affect your daily function. You need good dynamic flexibility to squat and pick something up off the floor, to reach into the backseat of your car, or to hop across a puddle. By exercising in proper alignment, you are dynamically stretching your tight structures and affecting how your brain is recruiting these muscles (neuromuscular response). A well-rounded fitness program is comprised of both dynamic and static flexibility training. Static flexibility is how the muscles lengthen across the joints at rest and it is a prerequisite for good dynamic flexibility. A split or a backbend are examples of extreme static flexibility. This chapter focuses on static flexibility training while maintaining good alignment. By stretching in good alignment, you ensure that you are targeting the correct structure.

Some people think that if they have never injured themselves, their bodies must be doing okay; they can continue jogging or playing soccer without much worry. However, as discussed in Chapter 3, most injuries are the result of repetitive microtrauma. Just because you have not experienced an injury does not mean that you will never have one. It just means that a potential injury has not yet reached your pain threshold. If you continue to function in an abnormal alignment with defined flexibility deficits, you will at some point sustain an injury. And, as most "worry-free" athletes discover

sooner or later, it is easier to prevent an injury than to rehabilitate one.

But injury prevention is not the only reason you should perform flexibility training. Other benefits are improved performance and ease of movement. The more flexible you are, the more fluid your movements will become. The goal of the *Peak Performance Fitness* program is to improve the efficiency and ease of your movements. The more efficient the movement, the less wear and tear on your body, and hence the less chance of injury. With increased body awareness, strength, and flexibility comes an improved self-confidence that will radiate to those around you.

How Did I Get So Inflexible?

All of your muscles work as opposing systems. If one muscle bends a joint, then there is an opposing muscle that helps straighten it. Typically, an individual is tight in one direction of motion and loose in the other, but if the muscles continue to function in this pattern, the muscle imbalance is reinforced. This abnormal pattern then sets the individual up for an injury.

If you have a tight tendon and muscle, you run the risk of tearing the tendon and/or the muscle. A common example of this is Achilles tendonitis, which is attributable to tight calf muscles. If the tendonitis is not treated, microtears develop that cause the tendon to weaken and, in many cases, rupture. At that point the only intervention is surgery, which entails a long rehabilitation. In short, stretch your tight muscles.

On the other hand, if you have excess flexibility at a joint, you run the risk of spraining the ligaments surrounding the joint. An example of this was Sandi, a 40-year-old former dancer and avid yoga participant. Sandi was very proud of her flexibility, but she had begun to develop low back pain. After she came to see me, I determined that while Sandi's hamstrings and low back were indeed very flexible, her hip flexors were extremely tight. The movement analysis revealed that Sandi was not able to activate her abdominal muscles in the proper sequence discussed in Chapter 3. She also had the telltale below-the-navel pudge, which further verified her transversus abdominis weakness. As a result of these multiple factors, Sandi was essentially "cheating" every time she took a yoga class. She compensated for her tight hip flexors by picking up the excess motion in her low back, and her poorly coordinated abdominal muscles were unable to assist in stabilizing her spine. So every time Sandi took a yoga class, she was spraining the ligaments in her back. After performing hip flexor stretching and the Low Back Solution for several weeks, Sandi was able to return to yoga without any low back pain.

Focused Breathing

Proper breathing is vital to any flexibility program. Focused breathing enables you to relax into the stretches and sustain this relaxation throughout the stretch, which is very important. Clinically, almost all of my patients required some type of focused breathing training. Many of them were "reverse breathers," which means that they had altered the normal breathing cycle and were breathing inefficiently. David, the 55-year-old attorney mentioned at the begin-

ning of this chapter, was the classic "reverse breather." When I first met David, I was struck instantly by how labored his breathing was. He took short, shallow breaths while his shoulders bobbed up and down. As his activity level increased, this pattern quickened. This reversed breathing pattern was reinforcing David's rounded shoulder posture, which further exacerbated his neck and jaw problems. In fact, David learned that simply by altering his breathing he could lessen his pain. When he breathed using his old pattern, his symptoms worsened, but once he learned to use focused breathing, his symptoms dissipated.

To determine if you are a "reverse breather" like David, try this test. Lie on your back and place your hands on your navel. Take in a deep breath and note which direction your hands move. If your hands move upward and your abdominal region expands, then you are breathing naturally. However, if you hands move downward and your abdomen flattens, then you are a "reverse breather." Regardless of your breathing pattern, focused breathing will still increase the efficiency of your breathing and improve your flexibility training.

For most of us, breathing is an unconscious act. However, by becoming aware of your breathing you will gain instant insight into your body and mind because breathing often mirrors your emotional state. For example, when you are tense, your breathing may be short and choppy. On the other hand, when you are relaxed, your breathing is usually even and full. Focused breathing is a technique that brings your breathing to a conscious level so you can learn more about it and yourself. This new awareness will enable you to relax into the stretches and sustain this relaxation throughout the stretch, both of which are important skills.

Focused breathing is a simple two-step process. Lie on your back and place your hands on your navel. Step 1 is the inhalation phase. Inhale deeply through your nose and visualize the air entering every part of your body. Your abdominal region should expand upward and sideways, and your hands should move up toward the ceiling. Step 2 is the exhalation phase. Expel the air through your nose while simultaneously activating your core, the technique discussed in Chapter 4. If this is your first time, repeat this breathing pattern ten more times so that your body can memorize it. This is also a good way to focus your concentration at the start of each exercise session.

When stretching, the part of the breathing you should focus on is the exhalation. It is during the exhalation phase that you should deepen your stretch. For example, when performing the hamstring stretch, you should attempt to pull your leg closer to your body every time you exhale. The depth and length of your breath should intensify toward the end of the stretch. It is also important that with each exhalation you activate your abdominals. The exhalation should begin below your navel and travel like a wave toward your head until the air escapes out either your nose or mouth.

Your Notes:

··

··

··

··

··

··

··

··

··

··

··

Chapter 10

The Flexibility Training Solution

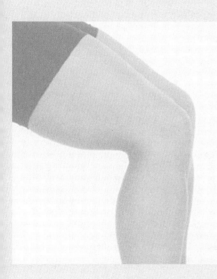

This is a comprehensive program designed to improve your static flexibility. The entire Flexibility Training Solution should be performed at the conclusion of every Cardio Solution session (discussed in Chapter 13). However, you should cross-reference each stretch with your postural evaluation from Chapter 2 and with your lifestyle to determine which stretches are particularly important for improving your alignment, and then perform those more frequently.

If you stand with your buttocks tucked underneath you (that is, if you look like you have no butt), then the hamstring stretch is very good for you. The tightness of this stance makes you vulnerable to hamstring strains and low back problems. Short hamstrings pull the low back into a flattened position, which predisposes an individual to a herniated lumbar disc. If you stand with your low back arched or sit at a desk all day, then the hip flexor stretch is excellent for you. Even the most flexible individuals tend to have hip flexor tightness. This is the stretch my patient Sandi (discussed in Chapter 9) used to alleviate her low back pain. Also, individuals with moderate transversus abdominis weakness should perform this stretch.

The quadricep stretch is good for everyone, especially if you suffer from knee problems. It is important to keep the knees touching during this exercise because you want to stretch not only the structures on the front of the leg but also the ones on the side (specifically the iliotibial band, as discussed in Chapter 5). However, if this stretch hurts your kneecap, discontinue it until your symptoms have subsided.

If you have a history of sciatica, an inflammation of the sciatic nerve, then the outer hip stretch is important for you. On the backside of your hip there is a muscle (the *pirformis*) that crisscrosses your buttocks. Your sciatic nerve passes either under, above, or through this muscle. Whenever this muscle tightens (which can often be a by-product of stress), it can reproduce the symptoms of sciatica. Sciatica can also occur whenever the sciatic nerve is pressed on by another structure, such as a herniated disc or because of arthritis. A symptom is typically a shooting or tingling pain down the leg. This stretch, which increases the flexibility of a tight pirformis, can also be performed while sitting and is also very helpful for individuals who stand with their feet turned out.

If you have a history of pain in your heel due to *plantar fascitis*, *heel spurs* (a bone protuberance in the heel), or Achilles tendonitis, or if you have flatfeet, then concentrate on the calf stretch. This is especially true if you wear high heels everyday. Wearing high heels on a regular basis will permanently shorten your Achilles tendon and calf muscles, predisposing you to a multitude of foot and ankle problems. Function over fashion—save your high heels for special occasions.

If you sit in front of a computer a lot, you should perform the chest stretch as well as the neck stretch every 2 hours. Tightness in this region of your body not only causes you to adopt a slumped posture, but also predisposes you to many neck and shoulder problems. If your postural evaluation reveals that one or both of your shoulders are elevated, then you should perform this stretch several times a day. People often have elevated shoulders as a result of carrying heavy bags or spending a lot of time on the phone. If you tend to carry a heavy bag with you at all times, consider purchasing a backpack with a waist strap. This allows you to distribute the load more evenly throughout your whole body. If you use the phone a lot, purchase a headset.

As with the previous exercises, you must make it so that your torso is visible when you do the flexibility program so you can monitor your alignment. See "What to Wear" in Chapter 4 for more information on this.

Equipment Checklist

■ A mirror to monitor your form.

■ Six-foot-long rope.

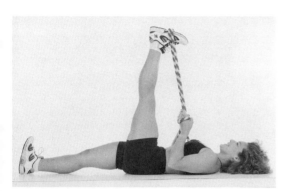

Hamstring stretch

Flexibility Training Solution Exercise 1

Hamstring Stretch

1. Loop the rope around your left foot.

2. Holding an end of the rope in each hand, lie on your back.

3. Press the back of your right knee toward the floor.

4. Activate your core and pull the left leg up and toward your body, keeping the knee straight.

5. Your neck should be long, with the shoulders relaxed onto the floor, and the back of the right knee should remain pressed into the floor.

6. Use focused breathing and hold the stretch for a count of 60.

7. Relax and then repeat once with the right leg.

8. You should feel a stretch in the back of the raised leg. If you do not, pull the leg toward your body until you do, always keeping the knee straight.

Check to Make Sure:

■ Chest is open and backs of shoulders are relaxed onto the floor.

■ Low back and back of opposite leg are anchored to the floor during the entire stretch. This ensures that you are isolating your hamstring muscle.

You Should Feel Work Going on In:

■ The back of the entire raised leg, from calf to thigh.

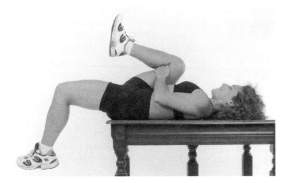

Hip flexor stretch

Flexibility Training Solution Exercise 2

Hip Flexor Stretch

1. Lie on your back on your bed, kitchen counter, dining room table, or anything that is high off the floor.

2. Slide your buttocks so that they are at the edge of the counter.

3. Pull both knees into your chest.

4. Activate your core and press your low back into the counter.

5. While keeping your low back pressed into the counter and your right knee pulled into your chest, slowly lower your left leg toward the floor until you feel a stretch in the front of your right hip.

6. Your neck should be long and your shoulders relaxed on the counter.

7. Use focused breathing and hold this position for a count of 60.

8. Relax and repeat once with the other leg.

Check to Make Sure:

- Chest is open and backs of shoulders are relaxed down.

- Your core is activated. Your low back must be pressed flat for this stretch to work.

You Should Feel Work Going on In:

- Abdominals.

- The front of your hip and thigh.

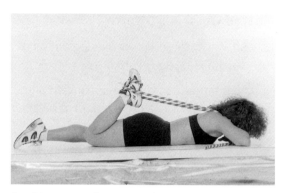

Quadriceps stretch

Flexibility Training Solution Exercise 3

Quadriceps Stretch

1. Loop the rope around your right ankle, holding one end of the rope in each hand.

2. Lie on your stomach.

3. Pull your right heel to your right buttocks using the rope. Try to keep your knees together during the stretch.

4. Use focused breathing and hold this position for a count of 60.

5. Relax and then repeat once with the other leg.

Check to Make Sure:

- Knees are touching.

- Shoulders are relaxed.

You Should Feel Work Going on In:

- The front of your hip and thigh.

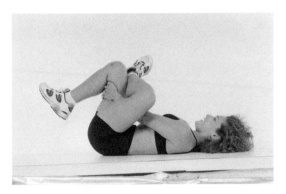

Outer hip stretch

Flexibility Training Solution Exercise 4

Outer Hip Stretch

1. Lie on your back

2. Bend both knees up.

3. Cross the left leg over the right thigh.

4. Grab the back of the right thigh and pull it toward your body.

5. You should feel a stretch on the outside of your left hip.

6. Keep your abdominals activated and your shoulders relaxed.

7. Use focused breathing and hold this position for a count of 60.

8. Relax and then repeat with the other leg.

Check to Make Sure:

■ Core is activated.

■ Shoulders are relaxed.

You Should Feel Work Going on In:

■ The outside of your hip.

Seated Outer Hip Stretch

1. Sit in a chair and cross one leg on top of the other leg as pictured.

2. Activate your core and lean forward until you feel a stretch in the outer hip region of the bent leg.

3. Use focused breathing and hold this position for a count of 60.

4. Relax and then repeat once with the other leg.

Check to Make Sure:

■ Core is activated.

■ Shoulders are relaxed.

You Should Feel Work Going on In:

■ The outside of your hip.

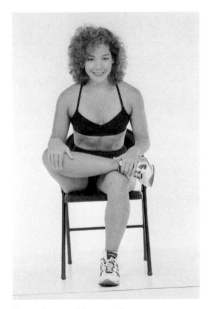

Seated outer hip stretch

Flexibility Training Solution Exercise 5

Calf Stretch

Upper Calf Stretch

1. Stand on the edge of a step.

2. Activate your core and relax your shoulders.

3. Drop your right heel off the step while keeping the knee straight.

4. Use your focused breathing and hold the position for a count of 60.

5. Relax and then repeat on the other leg.

Check to Make Sure:

- Core is activated.

- Knee of the leg being stretched is straight.

- Foot of the leg being stretched is neither rolling in or out.

You Should Feel Work Going on In:

- The calf.

Lower Calf Stretch

1. Repeat steps 1 to 5 of the upper calf stretch, except bend the knee of the leg being stretched.

Check to Make Sure:

- Core is activated.

- The knee of leg being stretched is slightly bent.

You Should Feel Work Going on In:

- The lower portion of your calf and the front of your shin.

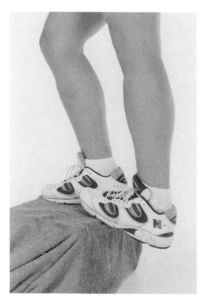

Upper calf stretch

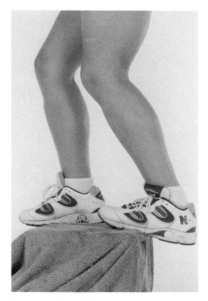

Lower calf stretch

Flexibility Training Solution Exercise 6

Chest Stretch

1. Stand facing the mirror.

2. Activate your core and relax your shoulders.

3. Bring your arms behind you and clasp your hands together.

4. Press your knuckles toward the floor.

5. Keep your chest open and navel in.

6. Use focused breathing and hold this position for a count of 60.

Check to Make Sure:

■ Core is activated and low back is flat.

■ Shoulders are relaxed back and down.

You Should Feel Work Going on In:

■ Chest and neck.

■ Upper arms.

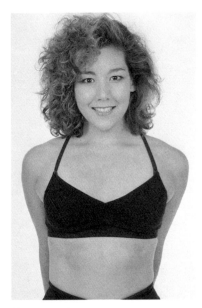

Chest stretch

Flexibility Training Solution
Exercise 7

Neck Stretch

1. Sit in a chair in front of the mirror.

2. Place your left arm in the small of your lower back.

3. Bend your right ear to your right shoulder

4. Gently press on the left side of your head with your right hand and bring your right ear closer to the shoulder.

5. Keep your back straight and your shoulders relaxed.

6. Use focused breathing and hold this position for a count of 60.

7. Relax and then repeat on the other side.

Check to Make Sure:

- Low back is flat and core is activated.

- The opposite shoulder stays in place (level) when the head moves.

- Mouth is closed.

You Should Feel Work Going on In:

- Neck.

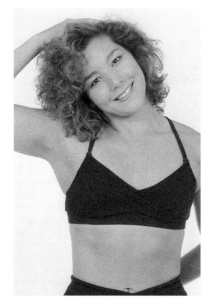

Neck stretch

Your Notes:

Chapter 11

Why You Should Fear Cardiovascular Disease More than Cancer

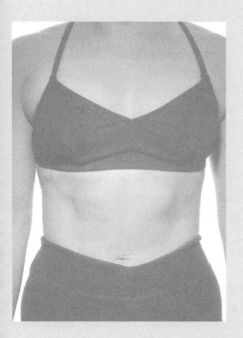

The harsh fact is, cardiovascular diseases are the No. 1 killer of women and men....Cardiovascular disease claims more lives each year than the next 7 leading causes of death combined—an average of 1 death every 33 seconds.

—AMERICAN HEART ASSOCIATION 2000
HEART AND STROKE STATISTICAL UPDATE

Think about it: If you add up the next leading causes of death in men and women—which are cancer, accidents, chronic obstructive pulmonary disease (asthma, emphysema, cystic fibrosis), pneumonia/influenza, and diabetes—they do not equal the number of people who die every year from cardiovascular disease. Most of these diseases are very serious but are often preventable through lifestyle management. For example, if you adopt a healthy heart lifestyle, you will also reduce your cancer risk.

Don't Only Senior Citizens Get Cardiovascular Disease?

According to the American Heart Association, approximately 17 percent of all the people who die of cardiovascular disease are under the age of 65. So, you might think, this means if you are under the age of 65, you should not worry much about cardiovascular disease. Wrong. Cardiovascular disease is progressive and its effects are cumulative. Signs of cardiovascular disease begin as early as your 20s. By the time a man reaches 45 years of age, his chance of having cardiovascular disease is approximately one in three. A 45-year-old woman's odds of having cardiovascular disease are almost three in ten. However, after menopause, the prevalence of cardiovascular disease evens out in both sexes, and women actually pass men after age 75. Furthermore, 80 percent of all individuals who suffer their first cardiac incident (*heart attack, chest tightness, cardiac arrest*) before age 65 die either during the incident or as a result of complications related to the incident. And of the individuals who die suddenly, 50 percent of the men and 63 percent of the women have had no previous symptoms of the disease. This means the first time you may learn you have cardiovascular disease is during your first attack, and there is a high probability that you may die shortly after learning this.

When I advise my patients about cardiovascular disease, many respond, "Well Jennifer, I gotta die sometime." Yes, we all die eventually. However, preventing cardiovascular disease is not about extending the quantity of your life; it's about preserving and improving the quality of your life. Immortality is a foolish goal, but emotional and physical wellness is an admirable one.

Anyone of us could recall a story, perhaps of a parent, friend, or loved one, that shows that cardiovascular disease is crippling and almost always ensures that you will spend the final years of your life dependent on medication, dependent on others, and in a steady state of deterioration. Cardiovascular disease robs its victims of their self-sufficiency and their ability to enjoy their lives.

So What Is Cardiovascular Disease?

Cardiovascular disease is any condition that affects the heart and/or the blood vessels. To understand cardiovascular disease, it is vital that you know how your body works. Imagine that your body is a vast distribution network where goods and services are exchanged. The heart is the central distribution center and the blood vessels are the pipes through which the exchange is carried out.

The heart is a large muscle located in the center of your chest. It is about the size of a clenched fist. Every time it contracts it sends blood throughout your entire body. The average person's heart at rest contracts seventy-five times per minute. This number is called your resting heart rate. This will be discussed in greater detail in the next chapter.

The *arteries* are the blood vessels that travel away from the heart. Arteries pick up oxygen and fresh nutrients and deliver them to your body's cells. This is the delivery pipeline for your body. The *veins* are the blood vessels that travel back toward the heart. Veins collect the waste products from the cells. This is the garbage collection pipeline for your body. The *lungs* are the central purification system for the whole network. It is at the lungs that fresh oxygen enters the blood and the waste product carbon dioxide is expelled. So every time you breathe you are bringing in a fresh supply of oxygen and ridding your body of carbon dioxide. There are other structures that help purify your blood, but a complete discussion of all these systems is beyond the scope of this text. Please see the bibliography for more in-depth reading material.

All four components—the heart, the arteries, the veins, and the lungs—must operate efficiently for good health. If there is an alteration in the function of one or more components, problems can occur. Most cardiovascular diseases begin with atherosclerosis, which is a blockage or hardening of the blood vessel walls. Early signs of this disease have been documented in individuals as young as 10 years old. These early sites are the precursors for sites of future blockage. Think of the pipes in your bathroom sink. If you let hair and other garbage collect in the pipes, then the sink will not empty quickly. If you continue to let this garbage build

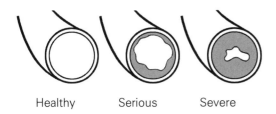

| Healthy | Serious | Severe |

11.1. Progression of blood vessel blockage

up in the pipes, there will come a day when your sink will not empty at all because your pipes are too clogged. Though this analogy is fairly simplistic, this is what happens to your blood vessels. But remember, your blood vessels do not get blocked overnight and multiple factors contribute to the problem. Below is a step-by-step explanation.

1. There is an initial trauma to the blood vessel wall. Certain risk factors can produce or make someone more susceptible to this trauma. Cigarette smoking, high blood pressure, high stress, viruses, and a family history in which a close blood relative has already had cardiovascular disease are examples of such risk factors.

2. The initial integrity of the tissue has been compromised by the trauma, and this spot becomes a ripe site for the deposit of fat. The more fat you carry in your blood (in other words, the more fatty foods you eat), the more fat you will deposit on your blood vessel walls. This is why it is important to know your cholesterol levels. Your cholesterol level is the marker of how much fat you have in your blood. More importantly, you should know what your levels are of high-density lipoproteins (HDLs) and of low-density lipoproteins (LDLs). HDLs are referred to as the "good" cholesterol, while LDLs are called the "bad" cholesterol. You want high levels of HDLs because they help transport fat out of your bloodstream. And you want low levels of LDLs because, due to their molecular design, they are prone to sticking to the blood vessel walls. Most physi-

cians recommend that your total cholesterol should be less than 200, while HDLs should be over 45 and LDLs under 130. If you haven't done so recently, get a blood test and see how you're doing.

3. If the damaging lifestyle is continued—whether it's a high-fat diet, cigarette smoking, a sedentary lifestyle, poor stress management, or all of the above—the blood vessel walls will be continually traumatized, more fat will be deposited, and then one day the blood vessel will become completely occluded (or blocked). A blood vessel usually needs to be 60 percent occluded before symptoms begin to show. This is why most individuals experience more symptoms of cardiovascular disease as they age. Older individuals have simply had more time to accumulate fatty deposits on their blood vessel walls. So if you are 25 years old, you can still have the early stages of cardiovascular disease; you just have not had enough time to pack on enough fat in your blood vessels to experience symptoms.

My Vessels Are Blocked...So What!

An occluded vessel is not a good thing. If a vessel is partially blocked, then blood cannot circulate efficiently through that area, which means that the cells on the receiving end of this vessel are deprived of oxygen and experience a build up of waste products. This affects the body's ability to heal and fight off infection in that area. This is why individuals with cardiovascular disease take longer to recover from

injuries or surgery and tend to get sicker more easily. If these cells continue to be deprived, they will eventually die. Many researchers believe that senility is less an aging issue and more an issue of poor circulation. They believe that the individual becomes forgetful because the brain is not getting an adequate supply of blood. This occlusion also increases the pressure within the blood vessels. This is called high blood pressure or hypertension.

Hypertension is one of the risk factors for cardiovascular disease and vice versa. One predisposes you to the other. Hypertension is defined as a blood pressure that is greater than 140/90. Most physicians recommend that you maintain a systolic (the top number) pressure less than 120 and a diastolic (the bottom number) pressure below 85. Remember, high blood pressure damages the blood vessel wall, which then predisposes the site to plaque or fat buildup. This plaque buildup increases the resistance to blood flow through the blood vessel, which increases the blood pressure. Also, having chronically high blood pressure can damage many of your body's organs to the point of failure. This vicious cycle cannot be addressed without major lifestyle changes. It is estimated that one in five Americans has hypertension, and 31.6 percent of them do not even know they have it.

Individuals with cardiovascular disease are also predisposed to blood clots. A blood clot is a collection of blood in the vessel wall. The danger of a blood clot is twofold. A blood clot can either grow to a size that completely closes off the blood vessel, or it can detach and travel to another location in the body, where it closes off another blood vessel. If this obstruction is long lasting, the cells around the blood vessel will die. A stroke is when a blood clot blocks off a blood vessel in the brain. All the brain cells that receive nourishment from that blood vessel die of starvation. Unlike other cells in the body, brain cells do not regenerate themselves. So once a brain cell is gone, it is gone forever. Since each brain cell has a particular job, a stroke patient loses the services provided by the dead brain cells. If enough brain cells doing similar jobs die, the individual loses the ability to perform that activity. This is why the outcomes of a stroke are so varied. One individual may lose the ability to speak, while another may not be able to walk or control his or her emotions. It's also why strokes are the leading cause of long-term disability in the United States. Strokes can often be fatal. In the United States, every 53 seconds someone has a stroke, and every 3.3 minutes someone dies from the complications of a stroke.

A heart attack is when a blood clot closes off a blood vessel in the heart. The damage is often irreparable and predisposes the individual to future heart attacks and heart malfunctions. Two-thirds of the individuals who suffer a heart attack will not make a complete recovery and approximately 31 percent (25 percent men, 38 percent women) will die within a year. A pulmonary embolism is when a blood clot blocks a blood vessel in the lungs. If not treated quickly, death can result.

While diabetes is not considered a cardiovascular disease, it usually coexists with it. Having one predisposes an individual to the other. Diabetes is a metabolic disorder that is the result of the body's inability to manufacture insulin, to utilize insulin, or both. Insulin escorts glucose, the main source of energy for your body, into cells. Without this escort, glucose just floats around in your blood while your cells go hungry.

There are two types of diabetes: Type I insulin-dependent diabetes mellitus and Type II non-insulin-dependent diabetes mellitus. Type I is when the body is unable to manufacture insulin because of the destruction of the insulin-manufacturing cells. The exact cause of this cell destruction is still unknown. Many researchers believe that it is a disorder with which some people are born. It is typically discovered during childhood. These individuals must take insulin shots for the rest of their lives.

While Type I diabetes is not preventable, Type II is. Type II diabetes is when the body's cells become resistant to insulin. The insulin tries to escort the glucose into the cell, but the cell does not let them enter. It is typically diagnosed after age forty and is always associated with obesity, a high-fat diet, and a sedentary lifestyle. Multiple studies have shown that by losing weight, decreasing fat intake, and becoming more physically active, diabetics are able to reduce the severity of their disease and in some cases rid themselves of it.

If diabetes is left untreated, it can lead to blindness, kidney failure, and loss of sensation in the limbs, which is the reason diabetics comprise a majority of all limb amputations. Furthermore, there is a cause and effect between diabetes, hypertension, and atherosclerosis. One predisposes the individual to the others, which means diabetics are prime candidates for heart attacks and strokes. The solution? Take care of your body.

On a Gentler Note

If this discussion of heart attacks, strokes, and death frightens you, it should. Your cardiovascular health is a very important issue. No one has ever died from tendonitis or back pain. More than 2,600 Americans die each day from complications of cardiovascular disease. However, the exciting news is that cardiovascular disease is preventable by making smart lifestyle choices, such as not smoking cigarettes, following a low-fat diet, maintaining effective stress management, and getting regular exercise. Furthermore, the lifestyle changes you make to prevent cardiovascular disease also aid in the prevention of cancer.

The next chapter, "The Cardio Solution," addresses improving your cardiovascular health through exercise. For further information on other lifestyle factors, see the resources listed in Appendix D.

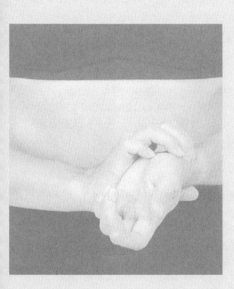

Chapter 12

The Cardio Solution

If I Had a Dime

If I had a dime for every time a student came up to me after an aerobics class and asked, "How many calories does this class burn?" I would be a millionaire. The reason this myopic view of exercise concerns me is because it ignores the primary purpose of cardiovascular exercise: to contribute to the improvement of your cardiovascular health. Note the word "contribute." Good cardiovascular health consists of regular cardiovascular training, a low-fat diet, and efficient techniques for stress management. This chapter focuses on improving the efficiency of your cardiovascular training, which includes determining your target heart rate and finding the best cardiovascular exercise for you. I also present a comprehensive walking program to get you started. For a more encompassing program of diet and stress management techniques, I highly recommend *Dr. Dean Ornish's Program for Reversing Heart Disease.* Dr. Ornish has spent the last 20 years researching how heart disease can be prevented and reversed through diet, exercise, and stress management.

Asking how many calories a class burns may seem like a harmless question, but in fact it masks a troubling underlying paradigm. Let us compare the individual who exercises to burn calories versus the individual who exercises for a healthy heart and lifelong fitness.

ARE YOU AT RISK FOR CARDIOVASCULAR DISEASE?

To determine your cardiovascular disease risk, please take the following quiz. Please check either yes or no.

You are a male over 45 or a female over 55.

☐ YES   ☐ NO

You have a close blood relative who had a heart attack.

☐ YES   ☐ NO

You have a close blood relative who had a stroke.

☐ YES   ☐ NO

You smoke or spend time in places with cigarette smoke.

☐ YES   ☐ NO

Your total cholesterol is over 240, or HDLs are under 35.

☐ YES   ☐ NO

You don't know your blood cholesterol.

☐ YES   ☐ NO

Your blood pressure is over 140/90.

☐ YES   ☐ NO

You don't know your blood pressure.

☐ YES   ☐ NO

You exercise less than three 30-minute cardiovascular sessions a week.

☐ YES   ☐ NO

If you answer yes to any of the questions, then you are at risk for cardiovascular disease. The more yes answers, the greater your risk.

So which one are you? Are you a calorie watcher or a healthy heart watcher? Most of us are somewhere between the two, having developed a mix of good and bad habits. However, if you find that your lifestyle closely resembles that of the calorie watcher, I recommend reading *Reinventing Your Life* by Jeffrey E. Young, Ph.D., and Janet S. Klosko, Ph.D. Often calorie-watcher behavior is a mask for other issues, such as depression, obsessive-compulsive behavior, or an eating disorder. While a discussion of these behaviors is beyond the scope of this book, if you find it difficult or impossible to change detrimental lifestyle habits along the lines outlined in this chapter, there may be deeper issues at work. For the health of your body and your spiritual well-being, consider finding a supportive environment and a qualified professional therapist to help. For further references, see Appendix D.

Five Simple Steps to a Healthy Heart

Here are the five simple steps you need to take to achieve and maintain a healthy heart.

- If you are a cigarette smoker, QUIT!

- If you don't know your blood values, get a physical and keep a copy of the results. Take note of your blood pressure and cholesterol levels. Your HDLs should be greater than 45 and your LDLs less than 130. The minimum number of physicals you should receive per decade should be as follows: two in your 20s, three in your 30s, four in your 40s, five in your 50s, and annual checkups after 60.

- If you are stressed out, get organized. If you are not in charge of your life, then who will be? I recommend using some type of calendar organizer (either paper or electronic) to help you organize your life. Also, seek out and learn healthful ways to manage your stress through meditation, exercise, yoga, or psychotherapy.

- If you are eating poorly, improve your diet. Read the books in the nutrition resource section in appendix D, and if necessary, consult a nutritionist for additional guidance.

- If you are out of shape, follow the guidelines below for developing a cardiovascular fitness program and begin the walking program at the end of this chapter.

How to Develop Your Own Cardiovascular Fitness Program

The only way to improve your cardiovascular fitness is by performing cardiovascular exercises in your target heart rate zone at least three times a week for a minimum of 30 minutes each session. Now, let us individualize the program to your specific fitness level. The best way to do this is to apply the FITT principle. FITT stands for Frequency, Intensity, Time, and Type.

Frequency

Studies have shown that you must perform cardiovascular exercises at least three times a week to achieve any benefits. Researchers have found that individuals who have active jobs and active leisure activities live the longest,

Calorie Watcher	Healthy Heart Watcher
Obsessively monitors the number of calories an exercise burns.	Monitors heart rate to ensure that he or she is exercising in his or her target heart rate zone (see page 100 for instructions on how to determine your target heart rate).
Recognizes food as a component of maintaining a trim figure. However, food becomes a constant temptation, and eating becomes a cycle of deprivation and bingeing. Since this individual is not eating healthfully, he or she is constantly looking for quick fixes to boost energy. Eating becomes a very stressful event.	Views food as a vital fuel for the body and is cognizant of the fact that if the correct foods aren't eaten, it affects his or her performance and sense of well-being. Also recognizes that all food is acceptable within moderation.
Since the ultimate goal is to be thin, this individual will pursue any means to achieve it. His or her lifestyle often includes cigarettes, excessive caffeine, drugs, or supplements—and anything else to "boost" his or her metabolism.	This individual recognizes that good health is a combination of factors. He or she lives in a way to minimize exposure to potential risk factors that might compromise health, such as cigarette smoke and poor diet.

while those with sedentary jobs and sedentary leisure activities have shorter lifespans. This does not mean you should quit your desk job and become a bicycle messenger. It merely means that when at work you should always choose physical options over mechanical ones, such as taking the stairs instead of the elevator or parking your car farther away from the office and walking. This also means that when it comes to your leisure activities you should incorporate some active ones into your lifestyle and always perform cardiovascular training at least three times a week.

Intensity

It is important to have objective measures to determine if you are exercising efficiently. The best objective measure is your heart rate. The intensity level of the activity you should perform will depend upon your fitness level and age, and so you must determine your personal intensity level.

Heart rate is the number of times the heart beats per minute. As discussed earlier, the average person's heart rate at rest is 75 beats per minute. The fitter an individual is, the lower the heart rate. Remember, the heart is a muscle, and the fit individual's heart is stronger and can send out more total volume of blood per squeeze than a less fit individual. For example, a typical endurance athlete, such as a marathon runner, can have a resting heart rate of 50 beats per minute. This means that the marathon runner's heart only has to squeeze 50 times to send out the same volume of blood as the 75 squeezes of the average individual. This principle holds true for your heart rate while exercising. A less fit individual's heart rate will

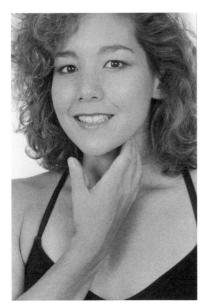

Finding your carotid pulse

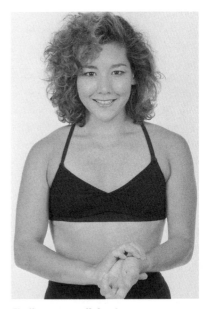

Finding your radial pulse

rise quickly, while a marathon runner's heart rate will rise, level off, and in many cases drop. The unfit individual's heart cannot keep up with the demand being placed upon it, while the endurance athlete's body is so efficient it actually needs added activity to maintain a high heart rate.

Finding Your Pulse

Before you can determine your target heart rate, you must find your pulse.

1. Place your first two fingers (not the thumb) at the carotid artery on your neck or the radial artery on your wrist. See the photograph on the previous page for further clarification.

2. Once you feel the pulse, count the number of beats for a whole minute. This number is your heart rate at that particular time. You can also count your heart beats for a portion of a minute (say, 15 seconds), and then multiply it (in this case, by four) to get your heart rate.

Time

Studies have shown that for maximum cardiovascular benefit you must exercise a minimum of 30 minutes at each exercise session. If you are new to exercise, you should review the walking program at the end of this chapter and follow the guidelines for new exercisers.

Type

The type of cardiovascular exercise you perform is very important. It should be something you like and an activity that you can perform on a regular basis. The following are specific recommendations for each fitness level:

If You Are New to Exercise

Walking is an excellent beginning activity for you. It is cheap, easy, and portable. Follow the sample Walking Program at the end of this chapter to get started. Before pursuing other cardiovascular activities, it is recommended that you be able to walk 30 minutes a minimum of 3 days a week within your target heart rate zone for at least a month. This will ensure that your cardiovascular and musculoskeletal systems are ready for a new activity. Once you are able to do this, then read the exercise suggestions for regular exercises.

If You Are a Regular Exerciser

First check to see if your current type of exercise is listed below under "Cardiovascular Activities." If it is not, determine if it qualifies as a cardiovascular exercise. To qualify, it must be an activity that exerts a continuous load on your cardiovascular system for a minimum of 30 minutes. Examples of activities that, of course, you can still pursue but that do not qualify are golf, tennis, basketball, hockey, and weight training. These are stop/start activities that do not exert a continuous load on your cardiovascular system.

If You Are an Elite Athlete

If you are a full-time athlete or compete regularly in a particular sport, you should purchase a heart rate monitor to measure your exercise intensity. Be judicious with its use and explore cross training, discussed below under "Cardiovascular Activities."

Determining Your Resting Heart Rate (RHR)

To determine your resting heart rate, you need to take your heart rate upon awakening three mornings in a row, then add these numbers together and divide by three. This establishes your average resting heart rate. Write your numbers below.

Day 1 RHR _____

Day 2 RHR _____

Day 3 RHR _____

Total _____

÷ 3 = _____ average RHR

Determining Your Target Heart Rate (THR)

To determine your target heart rate, you will need to do a little math. Make photocopies of this worksheet for future use and record your data on one of the photocopies.

$$220 \quad - \quad \underline{\hspace{2cm}} \quad = \quad \underline{\hspace{2cm}}$$
(your age) \quad (A)

$$(A) \quad - \quad \underline{\hspace{2cm}} \quad = \quad \underline{\hspace{2cm}}$$
(your RHR) \quad (B)

(A) represents your age-adjusted maximal heart rate; (B) represents the adjustment for your personal fitness level. Then determine 60 percent and 80 percent of (B). Studies have shown that for maximal cardiovascular benefit individuals must exercise at 60 to 80 percent.

$$\underline{\hspace{2cm}} \quad x \quad 0.60 \quad = \quad \underline{\hspace{2cm}} \quad + \quad \underline{\hspace{2cm}} \quad = \quad \underline{\hspace{2cm}}$$
(B) \quad (C) \quad (RHR) \quad (E)

$$\underline{\hspace{2cm}} \quad x \quad 0.80 \quad = \quad \underline{\hspace{2cm}} \quad + \quad \underline{\hspace{2cm}} \quad = \quad \underline{\hspace{2cm}}$$
(B) \quad (D) \quad (RHR) \quad (F)

220 – 35 = 185 (A); (A) – 72 = 113 (B); (B) x 0.60 = 68 (C); (C) + 72 = 140 (E). (E) is the lower end of your target heart rate zone. (B) x 0.80 = 90 (D); (D) + 72 = 162 (F). (F) is the upper end of your target heart rate zone. When you exercise, your heart rate should be somewhere between the two numbers, (E) and (F). You should check your heart rate approximately every 15 minutes to ensure that your exercise intensity is appropriate. If the number is too low, then pick up the pace; if it is too high, slow it down. In a couple of months as your cardiovascular fitness improves, you will need to recheck your RHR. If it has dropped, you should recalculate your THR and exercise in your new THR zone.

Cardiovascular Activities

Here is a list of common cardiovascular exercises. This is not an all-inclusive list, and any exercise that qualifies under the "continuous 30 minutes" rule can be considered a cardiovascular activity as well.

Speed walking

Running

Swimming

Bicycling (indoors or outdoors)

Rowing

Skating (roller or in-line)

Aerobic dance

Stair stepping

Cross country skiing

If you play a sport that doesn't qualify as cardiovascular exercise, begin with the Walking Program described below before moving on to a more intense activity. If the activity you are currently engaged in does qualify, then turn to Chapter 13 and learn how to integrate your cardiovascular work with the other programs in this book to create a new fitness program. However, the next time you perform your cardiovascular training, monitor your heart rate every 15 minutes to ensure that you are exercising in your target heart rate zone and vary your intensity level accordingly. Also, review the cardiovascular activity list to see if there is a second activity that you can pick up. Mixing and matching activities in this way is called cross training. Cross training is an excellent way to maintain interest, minimize injury, and consistently challenge your body.

Whatever your choice of exercise, your cardiovascular exercise program should meet the following criteria:

- **Frequency:** A minimum of three times a week.

- **Intensity:** 60 to 80 percent of your maximum HR.

- **Time:** A minimum of 30 minutes per session.

- **Type:** Start with walking, and then try other activities.

The Walking Program

Why walking? Walking is an excellent exercise and it requires minimal equipment. However, if walking is going to be your primary form of exercise, you should purchase a pair of walking shoes. These shoes are constructed differently from other sports shoes. Proper footwear is worth the investment because it will prevent injuries.

You should use the alignment cues you have learned so far and learn the following walking style to increase your walking speed. The best way to increase the intensity of your workout and ensure that you are in your target heart rate zone is by increasing your speed. The only way to increase your speed is by increasing the efficiency and pace of your arm and leg movements.

Perfecting Your Walking Style while Standing

1. Stand in front of the mirror in good alignment.

2. Bend your elbows to 90 degrees.

3. Continue to stand in place and swing your arms, emphasizing the backward punch of the elbows.

4. Check your form in the mirror and make the necessary adjustments, such as relaxing your shoulders, pulling your navel in, and opening your chest.

Perfecting Your Walking Style while Walking

Repeat steps 1 to 4 above.

1. Continue to swing your arms but begin to walk.

2. Notice that as the arm swing pace increases, so does the walking speed.

3. Check your alignment and make sure your heel is the first structure to hit the ground on each step.

Establishing Your Weekly Program

Beginning Exerciser			
Week	Frequency	Intensity (THR)	Time (in minutes)
1	3–5/week	40%–60%	10
2	3–5/week	40%–60%	12
3	3–5/week	40%–60%	15
4	3–5/week	40%–60%	18
5	3–5/week	40%–60%	20
6	3–5/week	40%–60%	22
7	3–5/week	40%–60%	25
8	3–5/week	40%–60%	28
9	3–5/week	40%–60%	30
10	3–5/week	40%–60%	30

After week 10, reevaluate your target heart rate zone.

11	3–5/week	60%–80%	30
12	3–5/week	60%–80%	30
13	3–5/week	60%–80%	30
14	3–5/week	60%–80%	30

Once you are regularly walking for 30 minutes while maintaining 60 to 80 percent of your THR, you can consider yourself a Regular Exerciser. Every couple of weeks thereafter, add 3 minutes to your total time, until you are walking for 45 to 60 minutes a session.

Regular Exerciser			
Week	Frequency	Intensity (THR)	Time (in minutes)
1	3–5/week	60%–80%	30

Once you have established the necessary pace for 1 or 2 weeks, every couple of weeks add 3 minutes to your total time until you are up to 45 to 60 minutes of cardiovascular exercise a session.

Elite Athlete

If you are an elite athlete or a long-time regular exerciser, I recommend that you use a heart rate monitor to measure the intensity level of your cardiovascular training for your specific sport. You can use the parameters set out in the Regular Exerciser section as a starting point. For example, if you are a tennis player, both running and bicycling are excellent cardiovascular training complements for your program. Outside of your regular tennis training, you should be either running or bicycling or doing both a minimum of three times a week at 60 to 80 percent of your target heart rate. Having a good cardiovascular base will enable you to outlast your opponent.

Your Notes:

Chapter 13

Choosing *Peak Performance Fitness* for Life

Here is a conversation I overheard in a local coffeehouse.

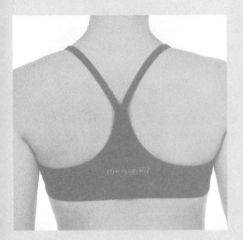

> *"Hey Jamie, how are you?"*
>
> *"I'm doing great! I leave tomorrow for a long trip."*
>
> *"That's wonderful. Where're you going?"*
>
> *"I don't know. I'm just going to get in my car and drive."*
>
> *"What do you mean you don't know where you're going? Aren't you going to take a map?"*
>
> *"I don't need a map. I'm just going to drive...."*
>
> *"How will you know when you've reached your destination?"*
>
> *"I won't. I just plan to drive...."*

While the above trip sounds very romantic, it isn't a very realistic approach to life. You wouldn't head off to college or buy a house without some careful planning to make sure you get the education or home of your choice. Even when it comes to vacations, most of us arrange things far in advance to make sure our limited time away is as relaxing and fun as possible. Why should we approach our health any differently? Your health deserves the same amount of attention and planning as any other aspect of your life. Good health ensures that you can enjoy all the different aspects of your life, such as career and family, with maximum vigor. Poor planning and inadequate goal setting are the reasons why most exercisers quit within the first 8 weeks of beginning a new program. They fail to approach exercise and their health systematically. Beginning an exercise program without well-defined goals or a schedule is like getting into your car for a trip without maps or a destination—you're as likely to arrive nowhere as somewhere, and your sense of success and accomplishment will be weak or missing. Through a simple three-step process, this chapter will help you develop an individualized plan for the next 12 weeks and begin integrating *Peak Performance Fitness* into your life. It will help you clarify your destination and create a map for getting there.

First, through a Personal Inventory you will determine why you want to exercise. Then, from that survey you will distill two specific goals. These goals will be written down and placed in locations for daily motivation. Finally, you will develop an action plan for implementing your goals. All of us need a reason to get up off the couch, lace up our shoes, and get moving. This chapter will help you determine *your* reason. Even if you are a regular exerciser or an elite athlete, this goal-setting exercise will help you focus your energy for maximum efficiency and results.

Here are some things to consider as you answer the questions on page 107. Feel free to review and revise your responses as you think of new things. Your response to Question 1 needs to be as specific as possible, because these statements form the basis of your goals. Why do you want to exercise? Is it because you cannot fit into an old pair of black jeans? Then write that down because that will be one of your goals—fit into black jeans within 12 weeks. If pain is your reason, then write down what activity brings on your pain. One of your goals may be to perform that activity without any pain. What made you decide to pick up this book?

For Question 2, your goals need to be objective. If your goals are not objective, then you will have no way of knowing if you have achieved them. An objective goal is one that is measurable and has a deadline. On page 109 you will find examples of general goals clients have submitted and their more objective versions. You should be able to distill two objective goals.

Your answers to Question 3 are the roadblocks you will need to overcome to achieve the goals set in Question 2. Thoughtful goal setting and a thorough action plan will help you overcome these obstacles. If you answer less than 5 hours for Question 4, then you need a reality check. For you to achieve your goals, you need a minimum time commitment of 5 hours a week. If you wrote anything for Question 5, erase it and throw your scale away. Your weight on the scale means nothing. In fact, you may gain weight during the program, since muscle is a denser tissue and weighs more than fat. A legitimate way to chart your progress is circumferential measurements of arms, legs, waist, and thighs. Since muscle is a denser tissue, as you add muscle, these numbers will fall, even when your overall weight remains steady. Question 6 is the image you want to visualize in your mind every time you exercise. This image is about more than aesthetics. It should include how you move and feel. The information for Question 7 should include both personal and professional commitments. We will use this information to design Step 3.

Step 1—Personal Inventory

1. What made you decide to exercise at this particular time?

2. List the primary and secondary goals you want to achieve by exercising.

3. "When I do not exercise as often as I should, it is usually because...." (*complete the sentence*)

4. How much time do you think you would need to invest per week in a sound exercise program? How much time are you realistically willing to invest?

5. Do you think you need to lose or gain weight?

6. Form an image in your mind of yourself in perfect physical condition. Now describe what you look like, how you feel, and so on.

7. List below your current time commitments throughout the week (see samples on pp. 110, 111)

Sunday	Monday	Tuesday	Wednesday	Thursday	Friday	Saturday

Step 2—Committing to Your Goals

Pick two goals from your responses to Question 2. They should be neither the most difficult to achieve nor the easiest. Make sure the two goals can be measured in objective terms, and review the goal setting exercise below if you need help with this. Then write your goals down on an index card and display the card where you will see it everyday. Calendars, computer terminals, bathroom mirrors, closet doors, and refrigerators are all excellent locations. You should read your goal aloud to yourself once a day. This will remind you of the commitment you have made to improving your health.

General Goal	Objective Goal
To get into better shape	Walk 1 mile in less than 15 minutes by the end of 12 weeks.
To have more energy	Get up at 6 a.m. every day and perform my *Peak Performance Fitness* program for 12 weeks.
To lose weight	Have waist and hips decrease by half an inch in the next 12 weeks.
To be stronger	Do 3 sets of 15 repetitions of bent knee push-ups by the end of 12 weeks.
To have better posture	Perform the Low Back Solution Exercise 1 with both my low back and neck flat on the floor by the end of 12 weeks.
To feel better about myself	Walk or run in a 5K race 12 weeks from today.

Step 3—Action Plan

Step 2 helped you determine your destination. The Action Plan will be your map for getting there. Review the table you completed for Question 7 (page 108) and note where there are gaps in your schedule. These openings will be your *Peak Performance Fitness* sessions.

Your *Peak Performance Fitness* program will consist of two components. The first component will be your strength and alignment program, which includes the Low Back and the Upper and Lower Extremity Solutions. Initially, these solutions will take you approximately 60 minutes to complete. The length of the session will decrease substantially as you become more proficient with the exercises and your form. Our goal is to develop a 45- to 60-minute strength and alignment program that you can perform two times a week. The second half of your *Peak Performance Fitness* program includes the Cardio and Flexibility Training Solutions. These solutions will take approximately 60 minutes to complete. The cardio portion can either be the Walking Program or a cardiovascular activity of your choice that qualifies under the FITT principle (see page 97 for more on this). The flexibility portion of the program will be the Flexibility Training Solution, which will take approximately 10 minutes to complete. All Cardio and Flexibility Training Solution training should be preceded by the Low Back Solution Exercise 1. This will "wake you up" and activate your abdominals so that you can maintain good form throughout the exercise.

Shown below is a sample schedule. However, if you find it too fatiguing to complete both the leg and the arm program in one day, you may alternate the days for each program. Your ultimate goal is to be able to perform all the exercises in one session, which frees up more time for cardiovascular training. On the following page is an alternate schedule. The first week focuses on the Lower Extremity Solution, while the second week emphasizes the Upper Extremity Solution.

Sample Schedule

Sunday	Monday	Tuesday	Wednesday	Thursday	Friday	Saturday
Rest and plan your schedule for the coming week	Low Back Solution Exercise 1 and Cardio/ Flexibility Training Solutions	Low Back and Upper and Lower Extremity Solutions	Low Back Solution Exercise 1 and Cardio/ Flexibility Training Solutions	Low Back and Upper and Lower Extremity Solutions	Low Back Solution Exercise 1 and Cardio/ Flexibility Training Solutions	Low Back Solution Exercise 1 and Cardio/ Flexibility Training Solutions (optional)
10 min.	*60 min.*	*45–60 min.*	*60 min.*	*45–60 min.*	*60 min.*	*60 min.*

Alternate Schedule 1

Sunday	Monday	Tuesday	Wednesday	Thursday	Friday	Saturday
Rest and plan your schedule for the coming week	Low Back and Lower Extremity Solutions	Low Back Solution Exercise 1 and Cardio/ Flexibility Training Solutions	Low Back and Upper Extremity Solutions	Low Back Solution Exercise 1 and Cardio/ Flexibility Training Solutions	Low Back and Lower Extremity Solutions	Low Back Solution Exercise 1 and Cardio/ Flexibility Training Solutions
10 min.	45–60 min.	60 min.	45–60 min.	60 min.	45–60 min.	60 min.

Alternate Schedule 2

Sunday	Monday	Tuesday	Wednesday	Thursday	Friday	Saturday
Rest and plan your schedule for the coming week	Low Back and Upper Extremity Solutions	Low Back Solution Exercise 1 and Cardio/ Flexibility Training Solutions	Low Back and Lower Extremity Solutions	Low Back Solution Exercise 1 and Cardio/ Flexibility Training Solutions	Low Back and Upper Extremity Solutions	Low Back Solution Exercise 1 and Cardio/ Flexibility Training Solutions
10 min.	45–60 min.	60 min.	45–60 min.	60 min.	45–60 min.	60 min.

Your Action Plan

Rewrite your schedule from the table in Question 7 into the table on page 112 and insert your *Peak Performance Fitness* program. On pages 113–115 are sample schedules for individuals of various levels.

Sunday	Monday	Tuesday	Wednesday	Thursday	Friday	Saturday

Sample Action Plans

Elite Athlete: Alex is the 28-year-old marathon runner introduced in Chapter 5

Sunday	Monday	Tuesday	Wednesday	Thursday	Friday	Saturday
11:30 a.m.– 2 p.m. Low Back Solution Exercise 1, 10-mile run, and Flexibility Training Solution	8:30 a.m.– 5:30 p.m. Work	8:30 a.m.– 5:30 p.m. Work	8:30 a.m.– 5:30 p.m. Work	8:30 a.m.– 5:30 p.m. Work	8:30 a.m.– 5:30 p.m. Work	Rest
3 p.m. Plan schedule for the coming week	6:30–7:30 p.m. Low Back and Upper and Lower Extremity Solutions	6:30–8 p.m. Low Back Solution Exercise 1, 3-mile run, 30-minute bike ride, and Flexibility Training Solution	6:30–8 p.m. Low Back Solution Exercise 1, 6-mile run, and Flexibility Training Solution	6:30–7:30 p.m. Low Back and Upper and Lower Extremity Solutions	6:30–8 p.m. Low Back Solution Exercise 1, 6-mile run, and Flexibility Training Solution	
	8 p.m. Dinner	8 p.m. Dinner	8:30 p.m. Dinner	8 p.m. Dinner	8:30 p.m. Dinner	

Regular Exerciser: Louise is the 44-year-old secretary introduced in Chapter 7

Sunday	Monday	Tuesday	Wednesday	Thursday	Friday	Saturday
9–10 a.m. Low Back Solution Exercise 1, 40-minute speed walk, and Flexibility Training Solution	9 a.m.–Noon Work	9 a.m.–5 p.m. Work	9 a.m.–Noon Work	9 a.m.–5 p.m. Work	9 a.m.–Noon Work	9–10 a.m. Low Back Solution Exercise 1, 40-minute speed walk, and Flexibility Training Solution
10:30 a.m. Plan schedule for the coming week	Noon–1 p.m. Low Back and Upper and Lower Extremity Solutions		Noon–1 p.m. Low Back Solution Exercise 1, 35 minutes on stair machine, and Flexibility Training Solution		Noon–1 p.m. Low Back and Upper and Lower Extremity Solutions	11 a.m. Family
11 a.m. Family	1:30–5:30 p.m. Work		1:30–5:30 p.m. Work		1:30–5:30 p.m. Work	
	6 p.m. Dinner					

New Exerciser: David is the 55-year-old lawyer introduced in Chapter 9

Sunday	Monday	Tuesday	Wednesday	Thursday	Friday	Saturday
9–11 a.m. Church	8–10 a.m. Partners meeting	6–7 a.m. Low Back Solution Exercise 1, 30-minute walk, and Flexibility Training Solution	6–7 a.m. Low Back and Upper Extremity Solutions	6–7 a.m. Low Back Solution Exercise 1, 30-minute walk, and Flexibility Training Solution	6–7 a.m. Low Back and Lower Extremity Solutions	7–8 a.m. Low Back Solution Exercise 1, 30-minute walk, and Flexibility Training Solution
Noon–1 p.m. Low Back and Lower Extremity Solutions 1 p.m. Plan schedule for the coming week	10 a.m.–7 p.m. Work	8 a.m.–7 p.m. Work	8 a.m.–6 p.m. Work	8 a.m.–7 p.m. Work	8 a.m.–6 p.m. Work	8:30 a.m. Family
1:30 p.m. Family	7:30 p.m. Dinner and family	7:30 p.m. Dinner and family	6:30 p.m. Kids soccer	7:30 p.m. Dinner and family	6:30 p.m. Church meeting	

The Peak Performance Fitness Weekly Exercise Log

The purpose of the Weekly Exercise Log is to keep you organized and motivated. The action plan is the map to your destination, detailing how you reach your goals. The Weekly Exercise Log is how you keep track of your progress; it lets you know you are going in the right direction. The *Peak Performance Fitness* Weekly Exercise Log should be placed in a three-ring binder and stored in your designated exercise space. (There are blank masters of all the *Peak Performance Fitness* forms in Appendix C.) Every Sunday, sit down and plan your exercise schedule for the week. This planning should include setting specific goals for each exercise session, such as weight and repetitions. If you don't plan it, it will never happen. The Sunday planning sessions should take about 10 minutes. At the end of each session, you should spend 5 minutes updating your Weekly Exercise Log. Keeping accurate records will help motivate you, since they will illustrate your progress as you become healthier and stronger.

Additional Tips

As discussed in Chapter 1, you need to find a place in your home and designate it as your exercise space. This will be the place where you keep your equipment, your Weekly Exercise Log binder, and your copy of *Peak Performance Fitness*. This space must remain free from clutter, be located away from the distractions of your home life, and always be available to you. This space is your personal sanctuary.

If you are exercising at the gym, you should have a designated gym bag that contains your copy of *Peak Performance Fitness* with one Weekly Exercise Log sheet tucked into the front and any equipment you may require that your gym does not have. Update your log at the completion of your workout prior to leaving the gym. Every Sunday review the previous week's log before placing it in your binder, and insert a fresh Weekly Exercise Log sheet into your gym bag. Developing simple rituals such as these will keep you organized and motivated.

Many people also find it motivating to exercise with friends. This allows them to have someone to share their progress with. However, determine if your potential exercise partner is as motivated as you are and has a similar exercise style and ability. You have enough roadblocks to overcome—your exercise partner should not become one of them.

What Happens after 12 Weeks?

When you complete your first 12 weeks, you should first reward yourself—whether by going out to dinner, buying a new exercise outfit, or otherwise marking the occasion. You have made it past the 8-week hump when most new exercisers quit. Then you should review your index card and determine if you achieved your two goals. If you did, congratulations! However, if you did not, then you need to determine why, since these roadblocks will not disappear on their own.

The next step is to reevaluate your goals and create a new action plan for the next 12 weeks. Reread the beginning of this chapter, complete Questions 1, 2, 3, and 7 of the Personal Inventory, and continue through Steps 2 and 3.

Sample Peak Performance Fitness Weekly Exercise Log for Alex

	Sunday	Monday	Tuesday	Wednesday	Thursday	Friday	Saturday
DATE	8/6	8/7	8/8	8/9	8/10	8/11	8/12
Low Back Solution 1	LEVEL 3	LEVEL 3	LEVEL 3	LEVEL 3	LEVEL 3	LEVEL 3	LEVEL
Low Back Solution 2	LEVEL	LEVEL 2	LEVEL	LEVEL	LEVEL 3	LEVEL	LEVEL
Cardio (min. 30 minutes)	Run 10 miles		Run 3 miles Bike 30 min.	Run 6 miles		Run 6 miles	
Stretches							
Hamstrings	✓		✓	✓		✓	
Hip flexors	✓		✓	✓		✓	
Quadriceps	✓		✓	✓		✓	
Outer hips	✓		✓	✓		✓	
Calves	✓		✓	✓		✓	
Chest	✓		✓	✓		✓	
Neck	✓		✓	✓		✓	
Lower Extremity Solution							
Straight leg raise	LBS / REPS	LBS / REPS 8/45	LBS / REPS	LBS / REPS	LBS / REPS 9/45	LBS / REPS	LBS / REPS
Sidelying leg lift	LBS / REPS	LBS / REPS 8/45	LBS / REPS	LBS / REPS	LBS / REPS 9/45	LBS / REPS	LBS / REPS
Wall sit	LEVEL / MINS.	LEVEL / MINS. 2/2	LEVEL / MINS.	LEVEL / MINS.	LEVEL / MINS. 2/2	LEVEL / MINS.	LEVEL / MINS.
Ankle eversion	LBS / REPS	LBS / REPS 8/45	LBS / REPS	LBS / REPS	LBS / REPS 8/45	LBS / REPS	LBS / REPS
Ankle dorsiflexion	LBS / REPS	LBS / REPS 8/45	LBS / REPS	LBS / REPS	LBS / REPS 8/45	LBS / REPS	LBS / REPS
Towel grabs		100			100		
Upper Extremity Solutions							
Sidelying external rotation	LBS / REPS	LBS / REPS 5/45	LBS / REPS	LBS / REPS	LBS / REPS 5/45	LBS / REPS	LBS / REPS
Push-ups (straight leg)	REPS	REPS 12/10/10	REPS	REPS	REPS 12/12/10	REPS	REPS
Dips (straight leg)	REPS	REPS 15/15/10	REPS	REPS	REPS 15/15/10	REPS	REPS
Facedown rows	LBS / REPS	LBS / REPS 5/45	LBS / REPS	LBS / REPS	LBS / REPS 5/45	LBS / REPS	LBS / REPS
Comments	Felt better	Put knees down during last push-up set	Run included 4 hills	Felt great!	Push-ups better 3rd wall sit 1-1/2 min.	Walked last 1/4 mile	

Afterword

This is the most exciting page of the book. Why, you ask? Because it is the beginning of your journey to having your best body ever. The reason I wrote *Peak Performance Fitness* was to empower you with the information and techniques necessary to take responsibility for your health and make permanent changes that will improve the way you look, feel, and move.

I firmly believe that people's sense of self-worth is tied to whether or not they feel that they have control over their life, and that this affects both their long-term physical and psychological health. You have always had the power, you just may not have had the information. Now you have both. You have the ability to not only create a better body but a better life. The clarity of vision and confidence that comes from having control over your body will spill over into every aspect of your life.

I ask that you reach out to others who you feel would benefit from the information in this book. By reaching out to others, you will in turn enrich yourself and recommit yourself to the goals you developed in Chapter 13. If you take care of your body, it will take care of you. I congratulate you and wish you the best on your journey.

Major Muscle Groups of the Front and Back of the Body

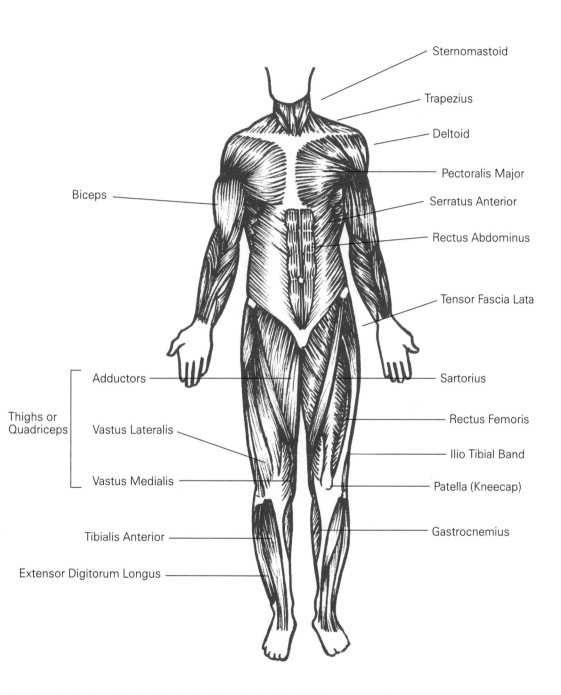

Sternomastoid

Trapezius

Deltoid

Pectoralis Major

Biceps

Serratus Anterior

Rectus Abdominus

Tensor Fascia Lata

Adductors

Sartorius

Thighs or Quadriceps

Rectus Femoris

Vastus Lateralis

Ilio Tibial Band

Vastus Medialis

Patella (Kneecap)

Tibialis Anterior

Gastrocnemius

Extensor Digitorum Longus

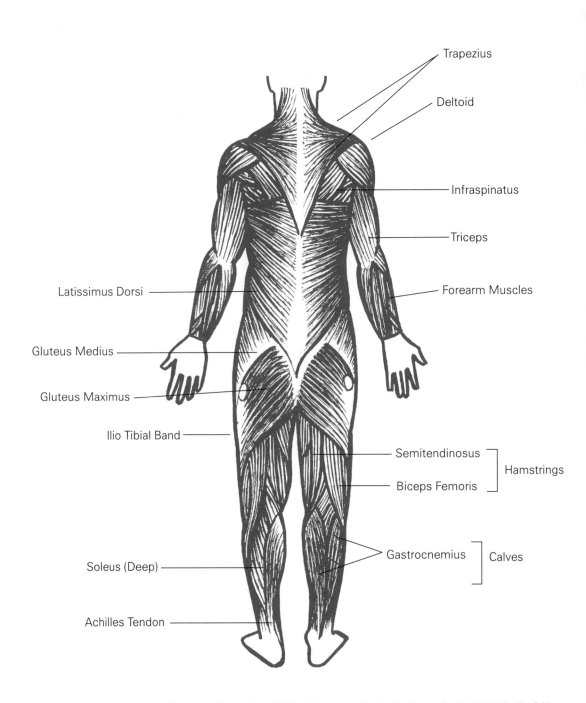

Trapezius

Deltoid

Infraspinatus

Triceps

Latissimus Dorsi

Forearm Muscles

Gluteus Medius

Gluteus Maximus

Ilio Tibial Band

Semitendinosus

Biceps Femoris

Hamstrings

Gastrocnemius

Calves

Soleus (Deep)

Achilles Tendon

Illustration reprinted with permission from *The Complete Guide to Joseph H. Pilates' Techniques of Physical Conditioning.* Copyright © 2000 by Allan S. Menezes.

Chapter 2

Sahrmann, S. *Diagnosis and Treatment of Movement-Related Pain Syndromes Associated with Muscle and Movement Imbalances.* Course notes, October, 1997.

Chapters 3 and 4

Ada, L., and C. Canning. *Key Issues in Neurological Physiotherapy.* Oxford: Bullerworth/Heinemann, 1990.

Cresswell, A. G., H. Grundstrom, and A. Thorstensson. "Observations on intra-abdominal pressure and patterns of abdominal intra-muscular activity in man." *Acta Physiol Scand* 144 (1992):409–18.

Cresswell, A. G., P. L. Blake, and A. Thorstensson. "The effect of an abdominal muscle training program on intra-abdominal pressure." *Scand J Rehabil Med* 26 (1994):79–86.

Cresswell, A. G., L. Oddsson, and A. Thorstensson. "The influence of sudden perturbations on trunk muscle activity and intra-abdominal pressure while standing." *Exp Brain Res* 98 (1994):336–41.

Hodges, P. W., and C. A. Richardson. "Inefficient muscular stabilization of the lumbar spine associated with low back pain: A motor control evaluation of transversus abdominis." *Spine* 21, no. 22 (1996): 2640–49.

———. "Contraction of the abdominal muscles associated with movement of the lower limb." *Physical Therapy* 77 (1997): 132–44.

Kendall, F. P. *Muscles Testing and Function.* 4th ed. Baltimore: Williams & Wilkins, 1993.

Moore, K. L. *Clinically Oriented Anatomy.* 3rd ed. Baltimore: Williams & Wilkins, 1992.

O'Sullivan, P., L. Twomey, and G. Allison. "Evaluation of specific stabilising exercise in the treatment of chronic low back pain with radiological diagnosis of spondylolysis and spondylolisthesis." *Spine* 22, no. 24 (1997): 2959–67.

———. "Altered abdominal muscle recruitment in patients with chronic low back pain following a specific exercise intervention." *JOSPT* 27, no. 2 (1998): 114–24.

Porterfield, J. A., and C. DeRosa. *Mechanical Low Back Pain: Perspectives in Functional Anatomy.* 2nd ed. Philadelphia: W. B. Saunders, 1998.

Strohl, K., J. Mead, R. Banzett, S. Loring, and P. Kosch. "Regional differences in abdominal muscle activity during various maneuvers in humans." *J Appl Physiol* 51, no. 6 (1981): 1471–76.

Chapters 5 and 6

Cerny, K. "Vastus medialis oblique/vastus lateralis muscle activity ratios for selected exercises in persons with and without patellofemoral pain syndrome." *Physical Therapy* 75, no. 8 (1996): 672–82.

Donatelli, R. A. *The Biomechanics of the Foot and Ankle.* 2nd ed. Philadelphia: F. A. Davis, 1996.

Doucette, S. A., and D. D. Child. "The effect of open and closed chain exercise and knee joint position on patellar tracking in lateral patellar compression." *JOSPT* 23, no. 2 (1996): 104–10.

Doucette, S. A., and E. M. Goble. "The effect of exercise on patellar tracking in lateral patellar compression syndrome." *Am J Sports Med* 20, no. 4 (1992): 434–40.

Fulkerson, J. P. *Disorders of the Patellofemoral Joint.* 3rd ed. Baltimore: Williams & Wilkins, 1997.

Graham, V. L., G. M. Gehisen, and J. A. Edwards. "Electromyographic evaluation of closed and open kinetic chain knee rehabilitation exercises." *Jour of Ath Training* 28, no. 1 (1993): 23–30.

Guten, G. N. *Running Injuries.* 1st ed. Philadelphia: W. B. Saunders, 1997.

Holmes, J. C., A. L. Pruitt, and N. J. Whalen. "Iliotibial band syndrome in cyclists." *Am J of Sports Med* 21, no. 3 (1993): 419–24.

Insall, J. "Current Concepts Review Patellar Pain." *JBJS* 64A, no. 1 (1982): 147–52.

Kendall, F. P. *Muscles Testing and Function.* 4th ed. Baltimore: Williams & Wilkins, 1993.

Kisner, C., and L. A. Colby. *Therapeutic Exercise Foundation and Techniques.* 2nd ed. Philadelphia: F. A. Davis, 1990.

Mann, R. A., D. E. Baxter, and L. D. Lutter. "Running symposium." *Foot & Ankle* 1, no. 4 (1981): 190–224.

Moore, K. L. *Clinically Oriented Anatomy.* 3rd ed. Baltimore: Williams & Wilkins, 1992.

Novacheck, T. F. "Running Injuries: A Biomechanical Approach." *JBJS* 80A, no. 8 (1998): 1220–33.

Saraniti, A. J. "The Effect of Prescribed Exercise Program for Chondromalacia Patella." Master's thesis, Richard L. Connolly College, Long Island University, October 1980.

Scott, N. W. *Arthroscopy of the Knee: Diagnosis and Treatment.* 1st ed. Philadelphia: W. B. Saunders, 1990.

Sutherland, D. H., L. Cooper, and D. Daniel. "The Role of the Ankle Plantar Flexors in Normal Walking." *JBJS* 62A, no. 3 (1980): 354–63.

Tiberio, D. "The Effect of Excessive Subtalar Joint Pronation on Patellofemoral Mechanics: A Theoretical Model." *JOSPT* 9, no. 4 (1987): 160–65.

Chapters 7 and 8

Andrews, J. R., and K. E. Wilk. *The Athlete's Shoulder.* 1st ed. New York: Churchill Livingstone, 1994.

Cailliet, R. *Neck and Arm Pain.* 3rd ed. Philadelphia: F. A. Davis, 1991

———. *Soft Tissue Pain and Disability.* 3rd ed. Philadelphia: F. A. Davis, 1996.

Glousman, R., F. Jobe, J. Tibone, D. Moynes, D. Antonelli, and J. Perry. "Dynamic electromyographic analysis of the throwing shoulder with glenohumeral instability." *JBJS* 70A, no. 2 (1988): 220–26.

Gross, M. L., S. L. Brenner, I. Esformes, and J. J. Sonzogni. "Anterior shoulder instability in weight lifters." *Am J of Sports Med* 21, no. 4 (1993): 599–604.

Hawkin, R. J., and J. C. Kennedy. "Impingement syndrome in athletes." *Am J of Sports Med* 8, no. 3 (1990): 151–58.

Kendall, F. P. *Muscles Testing and Function.* 4th ed. Baltimore: Williams & Wilkins, 1993.

Kibler, B. "Current concepts: The role of the scapula in athletic shoulder function." *Am J Sports Med* 26, no. 20 (1998): 325–37.

Kisner, C., and L. A. Colby. *Therapeutic Exercise Foundation and Techniques.* 2nd ed. Philadelphia: F. A. Davis, 1990.

Moore, K. L. *Clinically Oriented Anatomy.* 3rd ed. Baltimore: Williams & Wilkins, 1992.

Moseley, J. B., F. W. Jobe, M. Pink, J. Perry, and J. Tibone. "EMG analysis of the scapular muscles during a shoulder rehabilitation program." *Am J Sports Med* 20, no. 2 (1992): 128–34.

Townsend, J., F. W. Jobe, M. Pink, and J. Perry. "Electromyographic analysis of the glenohumeral muscles during a baseball rehabilitation program." *Am J of Sports Med* 19, no. 3 (1991): 264–72.

Chapters 11 and 12

Despres, J. P. "Visceral obesity, insulin resistance, and dyslipidemia: contribution of endurance exercise training to the treatment of the plurimetabolic syndrome." *Exercise and Sports Sciences Reviews* 25 (1997): 271–300.

Hillegass, E. A., and H. S. Sadowsky. *Essentials of Cardiopulmonary Physical Therapy.* Philadelphia: W. B. Saunders, 1994.

Jimenez, C. C. "Diabetes and exercise: The role of the athletic trainer." *J of Ath Training* 32, no. 4 (1997): 339–43.

Lee, I. M., and R. S. Paffenbarger. "Do physical activity and physical fitness avert premature mortality?" *Exercise and Sports Sciences Reviews* 24 (1996): 135–72.

McArdle, W. D., F. I. Katch, and V. L. Katch. *Exercise Physiology: Energy, Nutrition, and Human Performance.* 3rd ed. Philadelphia: Lea & Febiger, 1991.

McCance, K. L., and S. E. Huether. *Pathophysiology: The Biological Basis for Disease in Adults and Children.* 2nd ed. St. Louis: Mosby, 1994.

Ornish, D. *Dr. Dean Ornish's Program for Reversing Heart Disease: The only system scientifically proven to reverse heart disease without drugs or surgery.* New York: Ballantine Books, 1990.

Appendix B: Postural Evaluation Sheets

Front Postural Evaluation

Body Part	Proper Alignment	Your Alignment
Head	Centered over neck and shoulders	☐ Centered ☐ Tilted right or left ☐ Note asymmetry of the jaw ☐ Head protruding forward
Shoulders	Level without any forward rounding	☐ Level ☐ Right or left higher ☐ Both elevated ☐ One or both shoulders sloping forward
Hips	Level	☐ Place hands on top of hips and check if one hip is higher
Knees	Both kneecaps level and facing forward	☐ Legs are straight ☐ Knees touch when feet are apart (knock-knee) ☐ When feet are together, knees are apart (bow-legged)
Feet	Inside arch looks like a small dome Feet are parallel	☐ Inside edge of foot flattens out (flatfoot) ☐ High arch ☐ Foot and toes turn out (duck-foot) ☐ Foot and toes point inward while standing (pigeon-toed)

Side Postural Evaluation

Instructions: *Stand with your left side near the mirror. Repeat the evaluation with your right side near the mirror.*

Body Part	Proper Alignment	Your Alignment
Head	Ear over shoulder with slight curve forward of neck	☐ Chin held high ☐ Head protruding forward
Shoulder	Shoulder in line with hip	☐ Shoulder rounded forward ☐ Shoulder pulled back ☐ Marked rounding of upper back (kyphosis)
Abdomen	Entire abdomen is flat	☐ Flat ☐ Entire abdomen is protruding ☐ Upper abdomen is flat but lower portion protrudes
Knee	Knees straight	☐ Knee bent forward ☐ Knee bent backward
Hips	Slight curve in low back Hips in line with knee and shoulder	☐ Increased low back curve (lordosis) ☐ Flattened low back curve

Appendix C: Personal Inventory Sheets

Step 1—Personal Inventory

1. What made you decide to exercise at this particular time?

2. List the primary and secondary goals you want to achieve by exercising.

3. "When I do not exercise as often as I should, it is usually because...." (*complete the sentence*)

4. How much time do you think you would need to invest per week in a sound exercise program? How much time are you realistically willing to invest?

5. Do you think you need to lose or gain weight?

6. Form an image in your mind of yourself in perfect physical condition. Now describe what you look like, how you feel, and so on.

7. List below your current time commitments throughout the week.

Sunday	Monday	Tuesday	Wednesday	Thursday	Friday	Saturday

Peak Performance Fitness Weekly Exercise Log

	Sunday	Monday	Tuesday	Wednesday	Thursday	Friday	Saturday
DATE							
Low Back Solution 1	LEVEL	LEVEL	LEVEL	LEVEL	LEVEL	LEVEL	LEVEL
Low Back Solution 2	LEVEL	LEVEL	LEVEL	LEVEL	LEVEL	LEVEL	LEVEL
Cardio *(min. 30 minutes)*							
Stretches							
Hamstrings							
Hip flexors							
Quadriceps							
Outer hips							
Calves							
Chest							
Neck							
Lower Extremity Solution							
Straight leg raise	LBS / REPS	LBS / REPS	LBS / REPS	LBS / REPS	LBS / REPS	LBS / REPS	LBS / REPS
Sidelying leg lift	LBS / REPS	LBS / REPS	LBS / REPS	LBS / REPS	LBS / REPS	LBS / REPS	LBS / REPS
Wall sit	LEVEL / MINS.	LEVEL / MINS.	LEVEL / MINS.	LEVEL / MINS.	LEVEL / MINS.	LEVEL / MINS.	LEVEL / MINS.
Ankle eversion	LBS / REPS	LBS / REPS	LBS / REPS	LBS / REPS	LBS / REPS	LBS / REPS	LBS / REPS
Ankle dorsiflexion	LBS / REPS	LBS / REPS	LBS / REPS	LBS / REPS	LBS / REPS	LBS / REPS	LBS / REPS
Towel grabs							
Upper Extremity Solutions							
Sidelying external rotation	LBS / REPS	LBS / REPS	LBS / REPS	LBS / REPS	LBS / REPS	LBS / REPS	LBS / REPS
Push-ups	REPS	REPS	REPS	REPS	REPS	REPS	REPS
Dips	REPS	REPS	REPS	REPS	REPS	REPS	REPS
Facedown rows	LBS / REPS	LBS / REPS	LBS / REPS	LBS / REPS	LBS / REPS	LBS / REPS	LBS / REPS
Comments							

Chapter 4

Foam Roll

To order a foam roll, call 800-367-7393 or visit Orthopedic Physical Therapy Products' website at www.OPTP.com. Request OPTP foam roll 36 inches long and 6 inches in diameter, #FR366. The cost is approximately twenty dollars including shipping and handling.

Chapter 5

Orthotics

Most sporting goods stores sell Spencos. Or you can contact them at either (800) 877-3626 or at www.spenco.com to find the nearest dealer. Spencos typically cost less than twenty dollars. They run in whole sizes (5, 6, 7, 8), so I recommend you purchase a half size smaller than your normal size. For example, if you are an 8½, then you should purchase a size 8.

Chapter 6

Socks

Thorlo socks are not inexpensive. A pair can typically run around ten dollars. However, since they are so indestructible, you save money in the long run. Most sporting goods stores sell them, or you can call (800) 457-2256 for the dealer nearest you. The Thorlo website is www.thorlo.com. Wash the socks inside out so the reinforced bottoms stay fluffy.

Chapter 7

Occipivot

To order an Occipivot, call OPTP at (800) 367-7393 and request item #4502C. The Occipivot costs $39.50 plus shipping and handling.

Chapter 10

Healthy Cardiovascular Lifestyle References

Exercise

American Heart Association: www.american-heart.com

Glover, B., and P. Schuder. *The New Competitive Runner's Handbook.* New York: Penguin Books, 1988.

The Mayo Clinic: www.MayoHealth.org

Meyers, C. *Walking: A Complete Guide to the Complete Exercise.* New York: Random House, 1992.

Ornish, D. *Dr. Dean Ornish's Program for Reversing Heart Disease: The only system scientifically proven to reverse heart disease without drugs or surgery.* New York: Ballantine Books, 1990.

Nutrition

Clark, N. *Nancy Clark's Sports Nutrition Guidebook.* Champaign, IL: Leisure Press, 1990.

Hinman, B., and M. Snyder. *More Lean and Luscious.* Vol. 2. Rocklin, CA: Prima, 1988.

Ojeda, L. *Her Healthy Heart: A woman's guide to preventing and reversing heart disease* naturally. Alameda, CA: Hunter House, 1998.

Ornish, D. *Dr. Dean Ornish's Program for Reversing Heart Disease: The only system scientifically proven to reverse heart disease without drugs or surgery.* New York: Ballantine Books, 1990.

Stress Management

Moyers, B. *Healing and the Mind.* New York: Doubleday, 1993.

Sarno, J. E. *The Mindbody Prescription: Healing the Body, Healing the Pain.* New York: Warner, 1998.

Young, J. E., and J. S. Klosko. *Reinventing Your Life: How To Break Free From Negative Life Patterns and Feel Good Again.* New York: Plume, 1994.

Chapter 12

ANAD: National Association of Anorexia Nervosa & Associated Disorder

P.O. Box 7
Highland Park IL 60035
(847) 831-3438
www.anad.org

Distributes listings of therapists, hospitals, and informative materials; sponsors support groups and a crisis hotline.

Gurze Books
P.O. Box 2238
Carlsbad CA 92018
(800) 756-7533
www.gurze.com

A publisher that sells books and educational materials about eating disorders.

OA: Overeaters Anonymous
P.O. Box 44020
Rio Rancho NM 87174
(505) 891-2664

A twelve-step self-help fellowship; local chapters are listed in the telephone white pages under Overeaters Anonymous.

Index

Index

Index

impingement, 55
tendonitis, 55–56

S

Sacral region of the spine, 14
Scapula (shoulder blade), 57
Schedule
  fitness plan, 110–111
  pre-fitness program, 108
Sciatica, 80
Shin splints, 39, 42
Shinbones (tibia, fibula), 33
Shoulder
  bones, 57
  muscles, 58–60
Six pack, 17
Socks, 42
Spinal cord, 14–15
Spinal curves, 9
Spinal discs, 14
Spine, 14–15
  cervical region, 14
  lumbar region, 14
  sacral region, 14
  thoracic region, 14
Sprain
  ankle, 42
  definition, 14
Stress
  holding location, 52, 54
  prolonged repetitive, 2
Stretches
  calf, 85
  chest, 86
  hamstring, 81
  hip flexor, 82
  neck, 87
  outer hip, 84

quadriceps, 83
repetitive, 2
Stroke, definition, 93
Subluxation, 30
Sustained curl, 23

T

Temporamandibular jaw
  (TMJ), 52
Tendon, Achilles, 38
Tendonitis
  Achilles, 39, 75, 80
  biceps, 60
  definition, 31
  rotator cuff, 55–56
Tennis elbow, 53
Thighbone (femur), 33
Thigh muscles, 28–29, 35,
  37
Thoracic region of the spine,
  14
Tibia, shinbone, 33
Timing of muscle activation,
  13
TMJ. See Temporamandibular
  jaw
Towel grab, 50
Trauma
  acute, 14
  micro, 13

U

Upper extremity exercises,
  63–71

V

Vertebrae, 14

W

Walking
  cardiovascular exercise, 99
  muscle action, 30–32
Walking program, 101–103
  establishment, 102
Walking style, improvement,
  102
Wall sit exercises, 45–47

Y

Young, Jeffrey E., 96

THE COMPLETE GUIDE TO JOSEPH H. PILATES' TECHNIQUES OF PHYSICAL CONDITIONING

Applying the Principles of Body Control

by Allen Menezes, Founder of the Pilates Institute of Australasia

Almost 80 years ago, Joseph Pilates developed a bodywork system that is wildly popular today. Initially taken up by dancers and performers, his program focused on strengthening the core muscles of the abdomen and strengthening and increasing flexibility in the arms and legs. Today his techniques are practiced by celebrities such as Madonna, Vanessa Williams, Patrick Swayze, and Leonardo DiCaprio to maintain a sculpted but not overly muscular look.

Allan Menezes' guide to Joseph Pilates' techniques includes a complete floor program (no special equipment needed) that guides readers through basic, intermediate, and advanced routines, with detailed descriptions of each exercise and step-by-step photographs. There is a special section on relieving back, ankle, and shoulder pain, and insights on how the work can be adapted by athletes. Worksheets are provided to record progress, and an introduction gives the history and legacy of Joseph Pilates.

Comprehensive and precise, this book is for those who make feeling healthy and looking fit a way of life. Everyone—from new

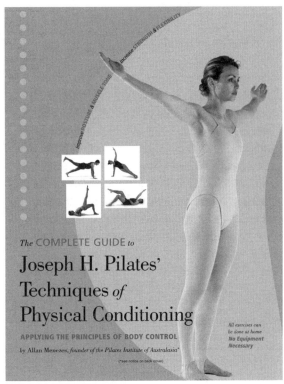

The COMPLETE GUIDE to
**Joseph H. Pilates'
Techniques of
Physical Conditioning**
APPLYING THE PRINCIPLES OF BODY CONTROL
by Allan Menezes, founder of the Pilates Institute of Australasia
(*see notice on back cover)

All exercises can be done at home No Equipment Necessary

208 pages ... 191 b/w photos ... 80 illus. & charts
Paperback $19.95
Spiral Bound $26.95

mothers to ballet dancers, from those with lower back pain to those who simply wish to improve their strength and flexibility—will benefit from this book.

Allen Menezes is the founder of the Pilates Institute of Australia and the Body Control Pilates Australia exercise studio franchise. He lectures internationally and conducts workshops and intensive instructor trainer courses for laypeople as well as healthcare professionals.

GET FIT WHILE YOU SIT

Easy Workouts from Your Chair

by Charlene Torkelson

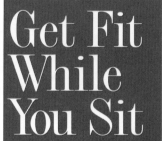

Get Fit While You Sit is a total body workout that can be done right from your chair, anywhere. It's perfect for office workers, travelers, and those with age-related movement limitations or special conditions. There are no complicated routines, no expensive gym memberships, and no equipment requiring a lot of space. You can even build these chair exercises into your daily home or office routine.

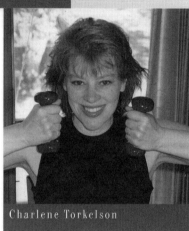

▶ *Low impact and fun*

▶ *A one-hour chair program including exercises for special conditions*

▶ *Bonus 10-minute workouts for computer users and the truly rushed*

The book offers three carefully designed programs. **The One-Hour Chair Program** is a full-body, low-impact workout that includes light aerobics and isolation exercises to be done with or without weights. A section highlights exercises for problem areas such as the back, upper legs, and stomach, and special conditions including arthritis and osteoporosis. **The Five-Day Short Program** features five complete, compact workouts for those short on time. Finally, computer users, travelers, and the truly rushed will enjoy the **Ten-Minute Miracles,** a group of easy-to-do exercises perfect for anyone at the office—even in a meeting–or on the go.

Each section includes clear directions and step-by-step photographs, and there is a checklist for monitoring progress. Written in a clear, encouraging, upbeat style, this is

160 pages ... 212 b/w photos
Paperback $12.95
Spiral Bound $17.95
Hard Cover $22.95

one program you'll stick with even if you've given up on others. No time? No space?

No excuses—just get fit while you sit!

Charlene Torkelson has been a dance and exercise expert for more than twenty years. She currently teaches a popular "chair class," and lives in Golden Valley, Minnesota, with her husband and three young children.

To order, or for our FREE catalog of books, please see last page or call 1-800-266-5592. Prices subject to change.

TREAT YOUR BACK WITHOUT SURGERY

The Best Non-Surgical Alternatives for Eliminating Back and Neck Pain

by Stephen Hochschuler, M.D.,and Bob Reznik, MBA

In this easy-to-read guide to back care and early treatment the authors—experts in the field—present non-surgical options for treating back pain, including:

- The four steps of first aid (ice, then heat—take anti-inflammatories—rest, but only for 2 days—as soon as you can, walk)
- an illustrated program of exercises that make the back muscles stronger and more flexible
- non-invasive treatments such as manipulation, physical therapy, and chiropractic
- alternative therapies like acupuncture, magnetic therapy, and tai chi

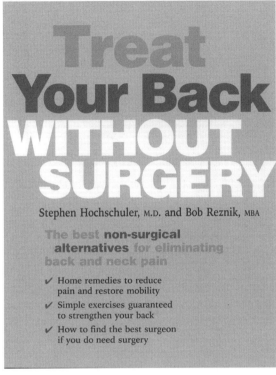

224 pages ... 47 b/w photos ... 6 illus.
Paperback $14.95
Hard cover $24.95

According to the authors, "virtually any non-surgical treatment that will not make you worse may be worth a try before you resort to surgery." Recognizing that surgery may be necessary at times, however, they offer guidelines on what to expect from diagnostic tests, how each type of surgery works, what kind of surgeon to choose, and how to find a good spine treatment center.

Stephen Hochschuler is a board-certified orthopedic surgeon specializing in spine surgery, co-founder and chairman of the Texas Back Institute and co-author of *Back in Shape*. Bob Reznik helped develop the Texas Back Institute Back Pain Hotline and currently runs Prizm Development, a company that works with healthcare providers to develop consumer friendly centers of excellence.

ORDER FORM

10% DISCOUNT on orders of $50 or more —
20% DISCOUNT on orders of $150 or more —
30% DISCOUNT on orders of $500 or more —
On cost of books for fully prepaid orders

NAME

ADDRESS

CITY/STATE   ZIP/POSTCODE

PHONE   COUNTRY (outside of U.S.)

TITLE	QTY	PRICE	TOTAL
Peak Performance Fitness (paperback)	@	$14.95	
Peak Performance Fitness (hard cover)	@	$24.95	

Prices subject to change without notice

Please list other titles below:

	@	$	
	@	$	
	@	$	
	@	$	
	@	$	
	@	$	
	@	$	

Check here to receive our book catalog ☐   FREE

Shipping Costs:
First book: $3.00 by book post ($4.50 by UPS, Priority Mail, or to ship outside the U.S.)
Each additional book: $1.00
For rush orders and bulk shipments call us at (800) 266-5592

TOTAL   _____
Less discount @_____%   (_____)
TOTAL COST OF BOOKS   _____
Calif. residents add sales tax _____
Shipping & handling   _____
TOTAL ENCLOSED   _____
Please pay in U.S. funds only

☐ Check ☐ Money Order ☐ Visa ☐ Mastercard ☐ Discover

Card # _____ Exp. date_____

Signature _____

Complete and mail to:
Hunter House Inc., Publishers
PO Box 2914, Alameda CA 94501-0914
Orders: (800) 266-5592   email: ordering@hunterhouse.com
Phone (510) 865-5282 Fax (510) 865-4295
☐ Check here to receive our book catalog

PPF 8/00